CAPTAINS OF CRUSH® GRIPPERS:
WHAT THEY ARE AND HOW TO CLOSE THEM
SECOND EDITION

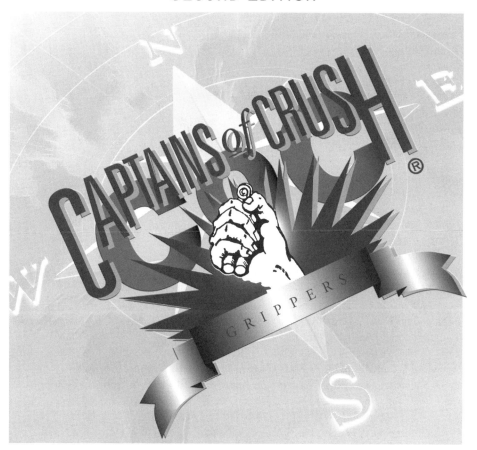

RANDALL J. STROSSEN, PH.D.
WITH J. B. KINNEY AND NATHAN HOLLE

IronMind Enterprises, Inc.
Nevada City, California

All rights reserved. No part of this book may be reproduced or transmitted in any form or by any means without written permission, except in the case of brief quotations embodied in articles or reviews. For further information, contact the publisher.

Captains of Crush® Grippers: What They Are and How to Close Them, Second Edition by Randall J. Strossen, Ph.D., with J. B. Kinney and Nathan Holle

© 2003, 2009 by IronMind Enterprises, Inc.
All rights reserved. First edition 2003
Second edition 2009

Cataloging in Publication Data

Strossen, Randall J., Ph.D.
Kinney, J. B.
Holle, Nathan

Captains of crush grippers: what they are and how to close them, second edition

1. Weight training   2. Fitness and health   I. Title
2009   796.41   Library of Congress Control Number: 2009928708
978-0-926888-84-5

Published in the United States of America
IronMind Enterprises, Inc., P.O. Box 1228, Nevada City, CA 95959 USA

Book and cover design by
Tony Agpoon, Sausalito, California

IronMind®, Captains of Crush®, Crushed-to-Dust!®, MILO®, Just Protein®, Super Squats®, and Rolling Thunder® are registered trademarks of IronMind Enterprises, Inc.

CoC, Guide, Sport, Trainer, No. 1, No. 1.5, No. 2, No. 2.5, No. 3, No. 3.5, No. 4, CoCG, CoCS, CoCT, CoC1, CoC1.5, CoC2, CoC2.5, CoC3, CoC3.5 and CoC4 are trademarks of IronMind Enterprises, Inc.

Photos of J. B. Kinney and his equipment by J. B. Kinney Jr., except where noted; photos in Chapter 6 courtesy of Nathan Holle; all other photos by Randall J. Strossen.

"It's not a crush . . . it's an obsession."
(Anon.)

If that's how you feel, this book is for you.

Other IronMind Enterprises, Inc. publications:

SUPER SQUATS: How to Gain 30 Pounds of Muscle in 6 Weeks by Randall J. Strossen, Ph.D.

IronMind: Stronger Minds, Stronger Bodies by Randall J. Strossen, Ph.D.

MILO: A Journal for Serious Strength Athletes, Randall J. Strossen, Ph.D., Publisher and Editor-in-chief

Paul Anderson: The Mightiest Minister by Randall J. Strossen, Ph.D.

Winning Ways: How to Succeed In the Gym and Out by Randall J. Strossen, Ph.D.

The Complete Keys to Progress by John McCallum, edited by Randall J. Strossen, Ph.D.

Mastery of Hand Strength, Revised Edition by John Brookfield

Training with Cables for Strength by John Brookfield

The Grip Master's Manual by John Brookfield

Powerlifting Basics, Texas-style: The Adventures of Lope Delk by Paul Kelso

Of Stones and Strength by Steve Jeck and Peter Martin

Sons of Samson, Volume 2 Profiles by David Webster, OBE

Rock Iron Steel: The Book of Strength by Steve Justa

Louis Cyr: Amazing Canadian by Ben Weider, C.M.

Bodyweight Exercises for Extraordinary Strength by Brad Johnson

The Complete Sandbag Training Course by Brian Jones

Conditioning Handbook: Getting in Top Shape by Brian Jones, M.S.

Grappling Basics: A New Twist on Conditioning by Brian Jones, M.S.

To order additional copies of *Captains of Crush® Grippers: What They Are and How to Close Them, Second Edition* or for a catalog of IronMind Enterprises, Inc. publications and products, please contact:

> **IronMind Enterprises, Inc.**
> P.O. Box 1228
> Nevada City, CA 95959 USA
> t – 530-272-3579
> f – 530-272-3095
> website: www.ironmind.com
> e-mail: sales@ironmind.com

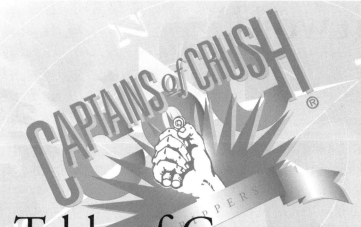

Table of Contents

Foreword		viii
Part I	**Captains of Crush® Grippers: What They Are** by Randall J. Strossen, Ph.D.	1
	Captains of Crush® Grippers: Packaging Timeline	2
	Captains of Crush® Grippers Family Tree	3
	Captains of Crush® Grippers: History in Highlights	4
Chapter 1	History: Family Roots and Evolution Toward Perfection	14
Chapter 2	Understanding Calibration: A Technical Twist	36
Chapter 3	Poundage Ratings: How Tough Is It to Close?	49
Chapter 4	Certification: World-Class Grip Strength	66
Part II	**Captains of Crush® Grippers: How to Close Them** by Randall J. Strossen, Ph.D., with J. B. Kinney and Nathan Holle	82
Chapter 5	Training Basics by Randall J. Strossen, Ph.D.	83
Chapter 6	Mortal Combat with the Captains of Crush® Grippers: How I Closed the No. 4 by J. B. Kinney	119
Chapter 7	The Holle Method for Training and Succeeding with the Captains of Crush® Grippers by Nathan Holle	154
Appendix 1	Gripper Myths and Facts	159
Appendix 2	Captains of Crush® Grippers: Rules for Closing and Certification	164
Appendix 3	Frequently Asked Questions about Captains of Crush® Grippers	168

Foreword

Hand strength has always held a unique place in the strength world—somewhat off in a corner, but also granted special privileges. Thus, grip specialists do not receive the attention of top lifters, but as the classic bodybuilding author John McCallum once observed, "The odd and pleasant thing you'll find is that gripping stunts are viewed by the general public out of all proportion to their actual difficulty . . . If you want a reputation as a strongman without going to too much trouble, a vise-like grip is the quickest and surest way to it."[1] Given many examples along this line—such as people who couldn't squat their way out of a wet paper bag but who have mastered tearing a deck of cards—it's hard to argue with McCallum's observation. Cheering fans and loyal admirers aside, though, the case for strong hands is easily made as there are many good reasons to pursue them.

In the days before barbells, a man's strength was measured by his mastery of unwieldy objects, many of which required an inordinately strong grip. Powerful hands were the natural byproduct of days filled with manual labor of many kinds. A day's work not only developed strong hands, it also created many natural opportunities to test or demonstrate one's grip strength.

As things progressed, the early barbells, dumbbells and kettlebells often had thick handles, partly of necessity since it wasn't possible to make them strong enough without using a lot of material, and partly to thwart those who tried to hoist them, since lifting something with a thick handle immediately turned the challenge into a test of grip strength. The bottom line was that having mighty mitts was vital if one were to succeed as a strongman.

---

[1] McCallum, John. *The Complete Keys to Progress*. IronMind Enterprises, Inc. Nevada City, California: 1993.

In recent years, the strength world was given a taste of this sort of challenge when, thanks to the efforts of John Staver, a replica Inch dumbbell went into production in 2000, with IronMind and Sorinex given the rights to sell it. Thomas Inch, a top early twentieth-century strongman, thwarted many a contender when pitting them against his thick-handled dumbbells. No matter how strong one's back or legs, if you couldn't hang onto the massive handle of the Inch challenge dumbbell, you weren't going to be able to lift it. What John Staver's replica did was bring this feat under the noses of modern-day lifters and strongmen, who couldn't resist testing themselves on this classic challenge.[2]

Even with the advent of highly efficient and wonderfully engineered barbells, one's hand strength can still limit what one can hoist on something that really is a test of overall body strength or power, not merely an isolated test of hand strength. Thus, for example, Olympic-style weightlifters use a hook grip because a conventional grip, let alone a thumbless grip, does not allow them to exert the full power of their legs and backs as they pull against the bar; and more than one deadlift—and title—has been lost because the lifter could not hang on to the bar. And for people who compete in modern strongman competitions, such as World's Strongest Man, a powerful grip is vital to one's game, so it should come as no surprise that some of the strongest hands around are not found in the circles of grip specialists, but rather on top strongman competitors. Similarly, for years we at IronMind have known that the ranks of Highland Games competitors include some guys with lethal grips.

The popularity of grip strength is also easily understood when one considers the breadth of its applications, from the ordinary to the life-preserving: you might need strong hands to open a jar in the kitchen, or they might make the difference between victory or defeat on the athletic field. In extreme cases, strong hands might define the margin between life and death in combat or in an adventure sport, such as rock climbing. The number of professions and vocations that benefit from grip strength seems almost limitless.

---

[2]When John Staver closed his foundry in 2006, production of the Inch replica ceased. Those who were fortunate to have acquired one should hang on to it—and those who want one will have to check the Internet or pursue other avenues.

Since its founding in 1988, IronMind has been at the heart of the grip world, and by the early 1990s we were recognized as the worldwide leader in the field: IronMind designs and sells cutting-edge grip training equipment; publishes the leading books on the subject; promotes the world's top grip people; and sponsors grip contests; and in recent years, we have been credited with spawning a minor industry based on the grip-related work we have been doing for the last two decades. The truth of the matter is that grip work, for all its seriousness, is also a lot of fun and we could not be happier that so many people have come to enjoy what used to be an underdeveloped and somewhat overlooked section of the strength world.

Even with the many grip training tools IronMind sells and the myriad reasons for being interested in greater grip strength, it's usually pretty simple to help someone who is starting off and only wants to buy one piece of grip equipment. Get a Captains of Crush® Gripper is what we recommend ninety-some percent of the time. That's how central they are to grip training, and because Captains of Crush Grippers also have a history, a set of traditions, and a following unlike anything else in their field, we felt it was time for us to roll up our sleeves and tell you their story—what they are and how to close them. The "what they are" section is perfect for everyone who wants to know from whence they came . . . we'll tell you some true stories and deflate some myths along the way. The "how to close them" part is vital because once you put a Captains of Crush Gripper in your hand, you'll be hooked on wanting to be able to close it, and for all its apparent simplicity, effective gripper training isn't always so obvious. For the latter task, crushing these beasts, we are going to step well beyond the usual sources of grip training advice, tapping into the experience and knowledge of top grip specialists as well as people with proven credentials in the larger world of strength. The result, we hope, will help you reach new levels of grip strength and in turn help others as well.

In the 1990s, everything under the sun lusted to be called an icon and the term became somewhat watered down through unwarranted use. Whether or not the guaranteed fifteen minutes of fame might have shrunk to fifteen seconds or merely the blink of an eye as more products vied for their moment in the sun, it's refreshing to know that not everything has the lifespan of a soap bubble on a windy day. Captains of Crush Grippers are one of the exceedingly few iron game products that have actually become an icon and established their enduring appeal. They are the gold standard of hand grippers and the universal benchmark for building and testing hand strength. They have inspired everything from Internet sites and me-too products, to the bonds of real flesh-and-blood friendships, and in these capacities, they have reached around the world. So powerful is their impact that IronMind has described Captains of Crush Grippers as "the gripper that changed the world." They have led to envy and jealousy, not to mention simple frustration and anger, but they have also created camaraderie and a sense of community, along with the loftiest feelings of accomplishment. And not content to stop in this lifetime, Captains of Crush Grippers have even caused changes in wills and altered burial instructions. That's quite a bit for something that weighs less than a pound and fits in the palm of your hand, but as we said, Captains of Crush Grippers are something very special.

Captains of Crush Grippers, available in ten strengths, are suitable for just about anyone, from the small and weak all the way up to World's Strongest Man winners—their ranks of devotees include everyday people and leaders in areas as diverse as government, sports and entertainment. And what all these people have in common is the burning desire, the passion, to squeeze the daylights out of a Captains of Crush Gripper.

Captains of Crush Grippers are used by people who are rehabbing injuries, seeking a firmer handshake, or wanting to improve in their favorite form of recreation, as well as those who know that their survival might depend on the strength of their hands. They have also served as a tool of redemption and as a means of developing a sense of self-efficacy: many are the people who have used a Captains of Crush Gripper to set goals, work hard, and then achieve what previously had been beyond their grasp. Sure, they closed a really tough world-standard gripper as a result of their focus and their efforts, but going far beyond that, they also developed a sense of self-worth and mastery that they carried forward into other facets of their lives.

Later in this book, you will read about the certification program IronMind developed in 1991 for our toughest grippers: being certified on the No. 3, No. 3.5, or No. 4 Captains of Crush Gripper grants elite status in the grip world. It's not within the reach of everyone, but anyone who achieves this level gains guaranteed recognition. IronMind has piles of intensely personal testimonials from people who describe their success with Captains of Crush Grippers as being among their biggest accomplishments, a driving force leading to their closest friendships and altering their lives. It's an amazing process, and this journey is available to everyone.

It's no wonder that people take such a deep and personal interest in Captains of Crush Grippers—their own grippers. So to all of you whose days are filled with hard work aimed at mastering these gems, and whose nights are filled with thoughts of succeeding beyond your wildest dreams, this book is for you.

As ever, train safely, wisely, and hard.

Randall J. Strossen, Ph.D.
IronMind Enterprises, Inc.
Nevada City, California

Part I

Captains of Crush® Grippers: What They Are

by Randall J. Strossen, Ph.D.

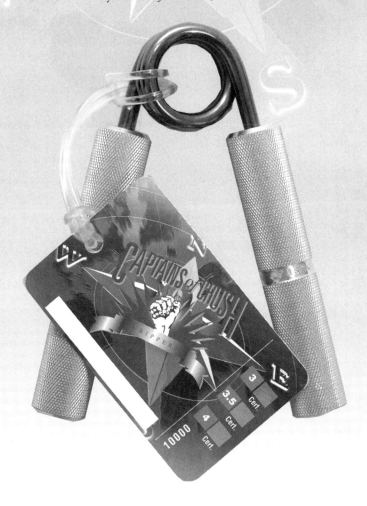

Captains of Crush® Grippers: Packaging Timeline

 1990 – wrapped in newsprint and numbered on outside with a black marker

 1991 – plain plastic bag, numbered with a black marker

 c. 1995 – Captains of Crush™ Grippers label on plastic bag

 c. 2001 – blue/grey diamond vacuum-sealed package with CoC logo

 2002 – rectangular vacuum-sealed package with CoC logo, blue border, with sports listed around edge

 2004 – rectangular vacuum-sealed package with CoC logo and two red stars

 2006 – rectangular vacuum-sealed package with gold CoC logo and shadow hand closing gripper

 2009 – blue rectangular vacuum-sealed package with CoC compass logo

Captains of Crush® Grippers Family Tree

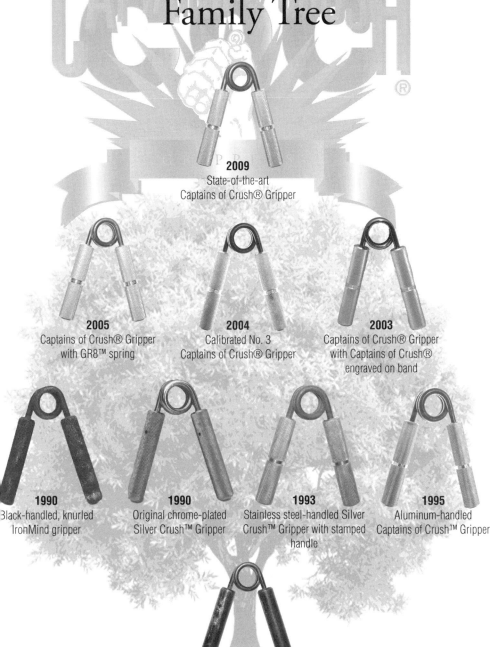

Captains of Crush® Grippers: History in Highlights

1964 — Iron Man grippers: Super Heavy Iron Man Grip Developer introduced
- made by Warren Tetting
- steel handles
- 3 strengths: "heavy duty," "extra heavy duty," "super duty"
- not standardized: variations in handle diameter, whether or not had knurling, and whether or not had keepers on the springs

1966–1967 — Randall J. Strossen buys an IronMan gripper (which he still owns), that was made by Warren Tetting

1977 — *Iron Man* magazine drops its grippers due to low sales

1988–1989 — While training for the World Wristwrestling Championships, Randall Strossen resumes grip training and contacts Warren Tetting, asking if he would like to make grippers for IronMind, just as he had in the 1960s and 1970s for Peary Rader's *Iron Man* magazine

Summer 1990 — reintroduction of Iron Man grippers by IronMind
- 3 strengths: #1, #2, and #3, all with knurled handles
- chrome-plated springs, painted steel, knurled handles; variations in color of handles (some painted grey, some black)
- made by Warren Tetting
- IronMind's print advertising campaign for its grippers begins in *Iron Man* magazine; it continues to this day
- IronMind begins work to improve the consistency and appearance of its grippers

Captains of Crush® Grippers: History in Highlights (cont.)

December 1990 — **Silver Crush™ Grippers introduced**
- continued improvements in accuracy, durability, and appearance
- chrome-plated mild steel handles and springs, uniform knurling pattern
- same 3 models as the first group: No. 1, No. 2, and No. 3
- made by Warren Tetting

1991 — **certification program established**
- Richard Sorin first person certified for closing the No. 3
- "Our Silver Crush™ Grippers are the most widely accepted standard for measuring crush strength . . ." (IronMind catalog, Volume 2, 1992, p. 9)
- offer lifetime warranty on spring

1992 — **John Brookfield becomes the second man in the world certified on the No. 3**
- Randall Strossen writes an article, "The Captains of Crush: The Men Who Know How to Get a Grip" for *IRONMAN* magazine, shining a spotlight on top gripsters, grip strength, and grippers in the mainstream bodybuilding/lifting world
- introduction of the Trainer Captains of Crush Gripper
- IronMind begins the development of a proprietary new spring
- experiment with lifetime warranty on the spring ends

1993 — **Silver Crush™ Grippers redesigned**
- all design and manufacturing operations are moved in-house
- "Starting with the heart of the gripper, we went to great lengths to develop a new, even more durable spring, one that has several times the life expectancy of the already super-tough spring we used last year." (IronMind catalog, Volume 3, 1993, p. 8)
- drift pin replaced with a high-tech, super-strength adhesive
- chrome-plated handles and springs replaced with stainless steel handles and natural steel springs
- clear band added at mid-handle as key element in trade dress

Captains of Crush® Grippers: History in Highlights (cont.)

- handles stamped with the abbreviation of the model name (e.g., T, 1, 2, 3)
- at the Yukon Jack National Armwrestling Championships, Cleve Dean crushes a No. 2 as easily as if it were a piece of paper
- publication of *MILO* begins, giving gripsters and grip strength the same exposure accorded to other strength sports
- poundage rating system developed: Trainer c. 100 lb.; No. 1 c. 140 lb.; No. 2 c. 195 lb.; and No. 3 c. 280 lb.

1994 — **introduction of the No. 4 CoC Gripper c. 365 lb.**
- "Our Silver Crush Grippers are the world standard for building and testing crushing strength, and are used by major league baseball stars and world champions from armwrestling to weightlifting." (IronMind catalog, Fall/Winter 1994, p. 6)
- "If you can fully close our No. 3 gripper with one hand, you will join the elite group known as 'The Captains of Crush™' and be a certified owner of some of the deadliest digits on the face of the earth." (IronMind catalog, Volume 4, 1994, p. 14)
- *MILO* (April 1994, Vol. 2 – No. 1) reports on longtime grip enthusiast and future Captain of Crush (CoC#3 – 2001) David Horne's 4th Goerner Grip Event
- Andreas Gudmundsson sees an IronMind gripper at the European Musclepower Championships (Callander, Scotland) and asks, "Is that a No. 3?", signifying the gripper's international presence

1995 — **Captains of Crush™ Grippers introduced**
- stainless steel handles are replaced by newly developed knurled, aircraft-grade aluminum handles
- continued improvements in precision, durability, and appearance
- IronMind publishes John Brookfield's book *Mastery of Hand Strength*; now in its second edition, the cornerstone in the field
- John Brookfield appears on the *Today* show as a result of IronMind's advertisement for his book *Mastery of Hand Strength*

Captains of Crush® Grippers: History in Highlights (cont.)

- "These grippers have become a legend in their own time—they are the toughest, best-crafted grippers in the world and are the accepted standard for testing and building the highest levels of crushing grip strength." (IronMind catalog, Summer 1995, p. 7)
- annual IronMind catalog presents a chart defining crushing, pinching and supporting grip, explaining the requirements for each (high, medium or low) for a number of sports; this launches a basic IronMind paradigm that will be widely adopted in coming years
- Ron Mazza, a game-changer from Bollenbach's Gym, certifies on the No. 3

1996 — **continued improvements in consistency, life and beauty**
- proprietary testing methods developed to ensure precision in manufacturing
- "No doubt about it: when most people think of grip strength, they think of what we call 'crushing grip,' what you use, for example, when you shake some one's hand, hard. . . when most people think of this type of grip, they also think about . . . sporting goods store grippers . . . Imagine this kind of gripper grown up." (IronMind catalog Volume 6, 1996, p. 11)
- IronMind publishes *Of Stones and Strength,* by Steve Jeck and Peter Martin. Steve Jeck vaulted the Inver Stone to new levels of awareness when he wrote to *MILO* about his world-changing meeting with this most famous of all manhood stones (January 1994, Vol. 1 – No. 4). Interestingly, Steve's letter included the comment, "I can confidently say that the *SUPER SQUATS* program and some grueling grip encounters with your No. 2 gripper played no small part in launching that load." (p. 2)
- Jay Lyttle certifies on the No. 3 and will later become the first "certified Captains of Crush to hit a hole in one!"

1997 — **Manfred Hoeberl certifies on the No. 3, a gripper he very nearly closed the first time he saw one**
- Joe Kinney certifies on the No. 3; Kinney had wanted a No. 3 the first time he ordered a Captains of Crush Gripper, but Randall Strossen told him to get a No. 2 instead; Kinney was right

Captains of Crush® Grippers: History in Highlights (cont.)

1998   Joe Kinney first to be certified for closing the No. 4
- Satohisa Nakada certifies on the No. 3 at 137 lb. body–weight, the lightest person to date to reach this distinction
- Jeff Maddy also certifies on the No. 3 at 518 lb. body–weight, the heaviest person to date to certify
- Jesse Marunde becomes "the first teenage Captains of Crush," certifying on the CoC No. 3 at 18 years of age
- Magnus Samuelsson certifies on the No. 3 CoC and wins the World's Strongest Man contest

1999   Joe Kinney closes a No. 3 Captains with two fingers, either hand
- Kevin Fulton, a Nebraska farmer who was in the vanguard of the grass-fed beef movement, certifies on the No. 3

2000   12-year-old Joe Kinney Jr. closes a Captains of Crush No. 1 gripper: "Before you cry 'unfair advantage' when you think about who Joe Jr. has coaching him, just remember that while his famous pa developed some unique training methods, they were all laced with a level of intensity that made failure an impossible action." (IronMind catalog, Volume 10, p. 14)
- Laine Snook certifies on the Captains of Crush No. 3, with World's Strongest Man winner Jaime Reeves as his official witness; Laine goes on to break the world record on the Rolling Thunder®, among his other top feats of grip strength
- Wade Gillingham and his father, Gale, the Green Bay Packer great, certify on the No. 3 Captains of Crush Gripper. Gale, at 55 years of age, is the oldest man at that time to achieve certification; Wade's big brothers, Brad and Karl, will certify on the No. 3 the next year
- John Wood certifies on the No. 3 Captains of Crush Gripper. Wood, whose father, Kim, had a three-decade career as an NFL strength coach (Cincinnati Bengals) got John started early: "I've trained on IronMind equipment since I was 12," John said.

2001   Kurtis Bowler certifies on the No. 3; Kurtis attended one of the very first CrossFit seminars ever held and his gym, Rainier CrossFit, was the eighth CrossFit affiliate

Captains of Crush® Grippers: History in Highlights (cont.)

- Derek Russell from Emerson Knives, a leader in the tactical knife market, calls Captains of Crush Grippers "the ultimate put up or shut up devices" (IronMind catalog, Volume 11, 2002, p. 30).

2002   Four of the Holle brothers—Nathan, Craig, Gavin and Jay—certify on the No. 3 Captains of Crush Gripper
- Wade Gillingham wins the IronMind St. Louis Steel Fingers Challenge as IronMind extends its support of grip competitions
- GNC begins the Blob Challenge at the Mr. Olympia; within two years, this will evolve into the GNC Grip Challenge, which uses Captains of Crush Grippers as one of its three tests of grip strength

2003   *Captains of Crush Grippers: What They Are and How to Close Them* by **Randall J. Strossen, Ph.D. is published**
- Close-the-Gap Straps are introduced
- Nathan Holle becomes the second man in the world to be certified on the No. 4 Captains of Crush Gripper
- IronMind publishes "Training With IronMind's Crushed to Dust!™ Grip Tools" by John Brookfield, who writes: "While the poundage listed can vary slightly, the Captains of Crush Grippers are amazingly consistent, accurate, and durable. These grippers have become popular around the world with strength athletes of all kinds, not only as a way to train your grip to the utmost but also to gauge or measure the strength of your grip." Brookfield also cites data from a hand dynamometer test, ". . . which shows that the ratings of these are grippers are well devised and right on target."
- Austin Slater certifies on the No. 3 Captains of Crush Gripper and contacts IronMind to make sure that his gripper really was up to snuff
- "The Captains of Crush Grippers are one of the most perfect products in existence," writes Kim Wood, strength coach, Cincinnati Bengals 1972–2003, and founding partner of Hammer Strength, a leading force in the Nautilus revolution (IronMind catalog, Volume 13, 2004, p. 31)

Captains of Crush® Grippers: History in Highlights (cont.)

- Captains of Crush Shield of Arms is introduced
- "Captains of Crush®" engraved on the clear band at mid-handle
- Magnus Samuelsson breaks the world record on the Rolling Thunder, the first man to both be certified on the No. 3 CoC and to have broken the Rolling Thunder world record
- on sight, Andrus Murumets breaks the world record on the Rolling Thunder; five years later, Murumets will certify on the No. 3 CoC
- David Erives, originally inspired when he read Randall Strossen's 1992 *IRONMAN* article on grip strength, certifies on the No. 3 CoC

2004 — **introduction of Guide (c. 60 lb.) and Sport (c. 80 lb.) models**
- benchmark No. 3 gripper is calibrated
- the "credit-card" rule is established in the certification program
- Magnus Samuelsson certifies on the No. 4 Captains of Crush Gripper
- Chad Woodall certifies on the No. 3 CoC
- Wade Gillingham consults with Randall Strossen and the GNC Grip Gauntlet is born; this most famous of all grip contests features Captains of Crush Grippers as one of its three elements testing the overall strength of one's grip
- GNC Grip Gauntlet appears at the Arnold Classic, the Show of Strength, and Mr. Olympia
- Captains of Crush Grippers sponsor the 2004 Arnold Armwrestling Championships

2005 — **continued refinement and accessory products offered**
- new GR8 springs used on all CoC Grippers
- CoC ID Card introduced
- Trevor Laing writes the "Captains of Crush" song
- Hand Gripper Helper introduced
- IMTUGs developed to complement Captains of Crush Grippers, part of what will become known as the Buddy System in gripper training
- Captains of Crush Grippers sponsor the 2005 Arnold Armwrestling Championships

Captains of Crush® Grippers: History in Highlights (cont.)

- The GNC Grip Gauntlet appears at the Arnold, the IHRSA Show, and Mr. Olympia
- ". . . you only as strong as your hands—it doesn't matter if you are wrestling alligators or going for the gold, if you can't hang on to whatever you're battling, all the core strength in the world won't do you one lick of good." (IronMind catalog, Volume 15, 2006, p. 39)
- CoC and the abbreviated model name (e.g., CoC 1) are added to the end of the handles

2006 — **introduction of "bridge" grippers: No. 1.5, No. 2.5, and No. 3.5**
- poundage ratings halfway between the Nos. 1, 2, 3, and 4 respectively
- Laine Snook breaks the world record on the Rolling Thunder, the second man in the world to certify on the No. 3 CoC and break the world record on the Rolling Thunder
- Captains of Crush Grippers sponsor the 2006 Arnold Armwrestling Championships
- GNC Grip Gauntlet appears at the FitExpo and the Arnold

2007 — **Richard Sorin re-certifies on the No. 3 Captains of Crush Gripper**
- CoC^2—Captains of Crush Compatible system is introduced for IronMind grip tools specifically designed to work with Captains of Crush Grippers
- in honor of Jesse Marunde, "the first teenage Captain of Crush," IronMind pledges US$500 to the educational trust fund for Jesse's children each time a teenager certifies on the No. 3, No. 3.5 or No. 4
- Captains of Crush Grippers named the official gripper of the Arnold Sports Festival, the GNC Grip Gauntlet, and United States Armwrestling
- Captains of Crush Grippers sponsor the 2007 Arnold Armwrestling Championships
- GNC Grip Gauntlet appears at the FitExpo, the Arnold, and Mr. Olympia

Captains of Crush® Grippers: History in Highlights (cont.)

2008
- Captains of Crush Grippers official website—www.captainsofcrushgrippers.com—is launched
  - "Are CoCs still made in the U.S. or have you farmed them out to Asia?" asks a customer. We reply, "Captains of Crush Grippers are made in the USA—always have been and always will be." (IronMind catalog, Volume 17, 2008, p. 55)
  - certification program expanded to include the No. 3.5 CoC Gripper
  - Tex Henderson is the first to be certified for closing the No. 3.5
  - CoC Key and CoC Caddies are introduced
  - Captains of Crush Grippers are featured in *The Sacramento Bee* and later in *Stanford* magazine
  - Captains of Crush Grippers named the official gripper of the World's Strongest Man contest
  - "Take the guesswork out of your grip training: Captains of Crush Grippers are the fastest way to a stronger grip" (IronMind Summer '08 flyer)
  - Captains of Crush Grippers sponsor the 2008 Arnold Armwrestling Championships
  - Captains of Crush compass logo design developed
  - Andrus Murumets certifies on the No. 3 CoC Gripper
  - GNC Grip Gauntlet appears at the FitExpo, the Arnold, and Mr. Olympia

2009
- Captains of Crush Grippers are featured in an article in *Business Week's SmallBiz* magazine
  - "Forging Strong and Healthy Hands around the World . . . If you have to pick just one grip-strength tool, this is it: Captains of Crush Grippers. . . . Nothing else puts power in the palm of your hand like a Captains of Crush Gripper." (IronMind catalog, Volume 18, 2008, p. 19)
  - Captains of Crush Grippers sponsor the 2009 Arnold Armwrestling Championships
  - GNC Grip Gauntlet appears at the FitExpo, the Arnold, and Mr. Olympia
  - *Captains of Crush Grippers: What They Are and How to Close Them* book revised

Please check for Highlights updates at www.captainsofcrushgrippers.com.

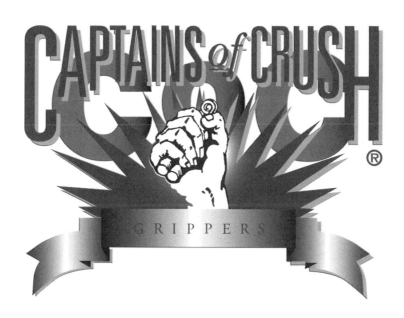

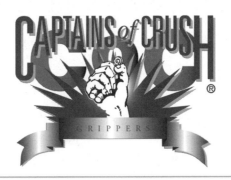

Chapter 1
History: Family Roots and Evolution Toward Perfection

Introduction

Captains of Crush Grippers are recognized around the world as the gold standard of grippers. They are the benchmark for building and testing grip strength, and officially closing the No. 3, No. 3.5, or No. 4 Captains of Crush Gripper is the most universally recognized measure of a world-class grip—impressive credentials by any stretch of the imagination.

The bug has bitten many people over the years and while most people are content to squeeze the daylights out of their Captains of Crush Grippers, other people like to examine them, talk about them, ponder their whys and wherefores, and discuss their history, features, and characteristics.

The Internet has brought such vast changes to the world that it's probably impossible to underestimate them, and while grippers—as wondrous as they are—are not at the center of the universe, they have been affected in profound ways by the worldwide web.

While the effects have been overwhelmingly positive, there have been some downsides as well: the principal negative influence the Internet has had on grippers and grip training is the spread of just plain false and even harmful information along with the facts, making it hard for the novice to sort things out. While Marshall McLuhan is correctly cited as the great mind who foresaw the "global electronic village," it was the crusty, cigar-smoking Mark Twain who in the nineteenth century noted, "A lie will be halfway around the world before the truth is even out of bed."

Thus, forums and boards without appropriate editorial functions can be hotbeds of misinformation about grippers, and we have heard many stories about IronMind's grippers—some true and some false. On a positive note, these same online communities can also be the meeting ground for gripper enthusiasts worldwide—places where information can be collected and shared, leading to bodies of knowledge and expertise available to all with a couple of keystrokes. Our intention is to contribute to the latter.

IronMind has been in this business since 1988, steadily immersed in our grippers. We fully understand the magnetism of these unique grippers, so we're here to tell our own story, addressing some myths and misinformation along the way, but primarily sharing basic facts as well as some colorful stories regarding Captains of Crush Grippers. Where we are now didn't happen overnight nor has the journey been an easy cruise down a well-designed highway: there have been some false starts, missed turns, and a few bumps and bruises along the way—but we are enjoying the ride and feel that we are living out our destiny.

Let's get started.

Advocacy since 1990

From its earliest days, IronMind has been the leading advocate of grip strength in general and grippers specifically. IronMind's roots go far deeper than even this, as I, IronMind's founder and president, bought in 1965 one of the earliest grippers that Warren Tetting made for the original *Iron Man* magazine, a rugged-looking beast of a gripper that I still own today.

One of the vehicles that IronMind has long used for supporting and developing interest in grip strength is its quarterly strength publication *MILO: A Journal For Serious Strength Athletes*. *MILO* covers such high profile events as the Olympics and the World's Strongest Man contest, as well as the world championships in a handful of strength sports, but it has also been distinguished by its inclusion of grip strength as a core content area. Not everyone has liked this, as we have had readers question why we would make note of "some guy closing a gripper in his basement"; or more broadly, critics might paint feats of grip strength as parlor tricks, not worthy of *MILO*'s finite resources.

Our counterargument is that grip strength, while not as central to one's overall training and performance as something like squats or power cleans, is important nonetheless, and more than one guy who takes the big lifts seriously has also enjoyed grip work as a sideline. And for our friends in armwrestling, for example, grip strength is as central to them as squats are to lifters. Additionally, grip strength is widely recognized as an asset in many sports and professions—everything from baseball to rock climbing—and might even save your life—consider adventure sports or law enforcement—so it's of no small concern to many practitioners.

IronMind began advertising its grippers and related grip equipment in 1990, and we have never stopped. It has been our pleasure to recognize the existing stars in the field, bringing them to the attention of a wider audience than had ever before been the case. In an effort to provide challenges to the growing legions of gripsters, IronMind began sponsoring grip contests in 2000, a practice we have continued to this day.

Roots

Original Iron Man grippers
Captains of Crush Grippers are the result of IronMind's dedication since the late 1980s to advancing—and trying to perfect—traditional nutcracker-

style hand grippers. Our goal then—and to this day—was to popularize what had been a tiny and short-lived cult item, as we also improved its looks, durability, and appearance. But first, it is important to recognize the pioneering role played by Warren Tetting, whose great contribution was making a nutcracker gripper that was super hard to close, turning it into a ballbuster, if you will.

Warren made the original Iron Man grippers that initially inspired me over forty years ago. These grippers were first advertised in the December 1964 issue of Peary Rader's *Iron Man* magazine as the "Super Heavy Iron Man Grip Developer," and I bought one shortly thereafter. Available in three models, called "heavy duty," "extra heavy duty," and "super duty," they were somewhat crude, and they varied in such features as the diameter of their handles, whether or not the handles were knurled, and whether the grippers had keepers on the springs. A far cry from anything you'd find in a sporting goods store, these grippers struck a chord with hardcore strength enthusiasts. As rugged in appearance as they were hard to close, the fact that they varied somewhat in appearance, geometry, and available strengths never really bothered anyone, and I am lucky enough to still have my original gripper.

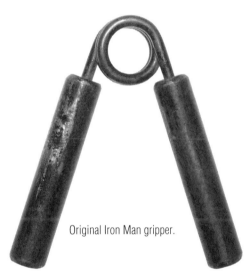
Original Iron Man gripper.

However, because the original Iron Man grippers had the confusing names "heavy duty," "extra heavy duty," and "super duty," and were unmarked, stories began to fly about who could or couldn't close which gripper. Thus began the fairly well-established practice of accidentally or intentionally misrepresenting the toughest gripper you had closed. One world champion powerlifter was well-known for walking around the warm-up room casually clicking an easy gripper and handing a really tough gripper to one of his competitors, challenging him with "Can you do this?" which of course he couldn't. The idea was that this warm-up room psych-out would carry over to competition platform performance.

Another powerlifter, this one of dubious repute, brazenly proclaimed that he had closed the toughest of all the old Iron Man grippers. One day he made the mistake of repeating this to a certain grip man, talking about the really tough Iron Man gripper he used to have, a gripper so tough that only he could close it. He went on describe what a pity it was that he'd lost the gripper. "No problem," the grip man replied, and pulled one of its cousins from his brief case. The spin doctor looked as if he had just swallowed a frog, and for a few minutes it became a case of shut the gripper or shut your mouth, your choice. Suffice it say that it was the mouth that closed when the gripper proved beyond the strength of the big talker.

Then, as now, tall tales mixed freely with the facts, but as long as nobody took the stories too seriously, everyone had a good time trying to close these grippers.

Early IronMind grippers
Those original Iron Man grippers might seem somewhat Neanderthal today, but if it were not for them, Captains of Crush Grippers are unlikely to have come into being. Also, while grippers of this general style date back about one hundred years, it was Warren Tetting who had the vision to make grippers suitable for the strongest people around.

In the late 1980s, after years of being a fan at the fabled Petaluma World Wristwrestling Championships, I decided to compete, and as part of my training I not only pulled out my old gripper, but as things developed, contacted Warren Tetting. The grippers that Warren made never hit the mainstream radar and had languished for decades, all but going out of production after Peary Rader quit carrying them in 1977 due to low sales—but Warren was still happy to make his grippers for those who wanted to buy them. IronMind did—and we put up the money to bring them back into production, and more than that, IronMind went on a mission to create a wider appreciation for grip training and grip strength, with grippers being a central part of our effort.

Not too much later, IronMind began selling what initially was a reintroduction of those old Iron Man grippers. Our earliest IronMind grippers were advertised as #1: "heavy duty"; #2: "extra-heavy"; and #3: "super-heavy," as we created the first significant element of our product's trade dress. Our numbering system was designed to give compact names that clearly showed the progression of one gripper to another.

Grippers like these are a specialty item, but even with their narrow market, we wanted other people to share our appreciation for them, so I began to write about them and to publicize the top grip guys of the day as we continued our close collaboration with Warren. We loved these things and even if nobody else shared our vision, IronMind felt that grippers could and should be more than they ever had been—luckily for us, some other people agreed.

Richard and John

It was in these earliest days of IronMind that I was introduced to Richard Sorin and, shortly after, to John Brookfield. Back then, the top tier of the grip world was almost completely defined by two names: Richard and John.

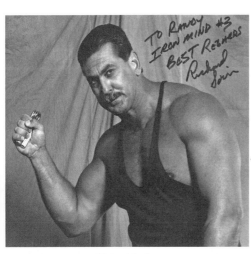

Richard Sorin.

Richard's secretary called me up in 1990 and said that her boss wanted her to order some of our grippers. Warren, it turned out, knew of Richard from his earlier exploits with grippers. I went on to write a number of articles featuring Richard's prodigious feats of hand strength, and between his ability and the exposure IronMind generated, Richard Sorin developed into the first modern-day grip strength star.

It's hard for people to appreciate this now, but back in 1991, Richard was the only person in the world we knew of who we believed could actually close our No. 3 gripper—and he was the first to say that he couldn't do it every time he tried. People, strong people who could manage a No. 1, for example, but were stymied by a No. 2 got goggle-eyed hearing that Richard could close a No. 3 IronMind gripper.

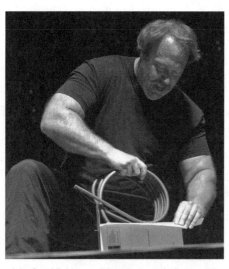

John Brookfield never faltered when winding up this 20' 6"-long steel bar at the 2005 *IRONMAN* Pro Bodybuilding contest.

John Brookfield called me up one day shortly after Richard had contacted us, and introduced himself by saying that he was a professional strongman and had the goal of developing the world's strongest hands, so he wanted to buy some of our grippers. Subsequently, John was also featured prominently in grip-related articles I wrote, beginning in the early 1990s. In the May 1992 issue of *IRONMAN* magazine, I had an article called "The Captains of Crush: The Men Who Know How to Get a Grip," and it talked about the exploits of Gary Stich, who had made something of a name for himself with his performances on plate-loaded grip machines; Richard Sorin, who was the best in the day on IronMind grippers and on pinch gripping; Steve "the Mighty Stefan" Sadicario, who did traditional feats of strength; and John Brookfield, who was our choice to win any decathlon of finger–hand–wrist exploits. More than ten years later, David Erives, a notable grip guy, told me he had read that article as a kid and that was what inspired him to take up grip training—he was amazed to read about what Richard Sorin could do and wanted to see if he could do likewise.

This was the beginning of taking feats of grip strength—and those who excelled at them—to new heights of public awareness and appreciation. To give you an idea of the extent to which IronMind was able to help elevate grip strength from a basement corner to the mainstream, John Brookfield was invited to appear on the *Today* show as a result of something I wrote about him in the 1995 IronMind catalog. John was the second person in the world IronMind certified on the No. 3 Captains of Crush Gripper, but what might surprise people is that he had anything but an easy time with it. Nonetheless, by pounding away at it, John conquered the No. 3 CoC and even though he has been at least semi-retired from specializing in this type of thing for years, John continues to be capable of impressive feats of hand and lower-arm strength.

Not limited to performing feats of strength, John Brookfield has gone on to write extensively about grip training, and his first book, *Mastery of Hand Strength*, has become the classic in the field. We feel that it is important to recognize that John—by virtue of his accomplishments, his incredibly fertile mind when it comes to training, and his prolific writings on the subject—is without a doubt one of the people who was most important and most influential in fueling the current interest in hand strength and grip training.

Silver Crush™ Grippers
Having started selling perfectly functional but arguably somewhat primitive grippers in 1990, IronMind introduced its Silver Crush™ Grippers shortly thereafter. Sometimes incorrectly referred to as being made from stainless steel, these grippers actually got their sparkle from their chrome-plated finish. They still had the heart and soul of their mighty forebears, and in some ways we might have been accused of

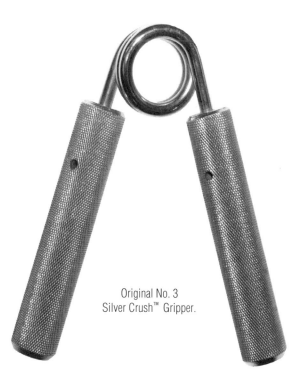

Original No. 3 Silver Crush™ Gripper.

gilding a lily, but we saw certain advantages in making these changes: it seemed as if the grippers we had been selling would only benefit from a getting a little dressed up. Incidentally, you might wonder what Richard Sorin thought about his then-new IronMind gripper? In September 1990, Richard wrote me: "Thank you so much for the #3 gripper. It is as nice as I could imagine . . . The pressure required to shut the gripper seems identical to the Iron Man grippers." This is more than a nice little colorful quote: it helps us introduce the somewhat slippery subject of just how hard it is to close a particular gripper or just how consistent a group of grippers might be.

The force required to close these grippers has always been somewhat mysterious if not contentious, and we'll talk more about the subject in a bit (see Chapter 3, Poundage Ratings: How Tough Is It to Close?).

As mentioned, because these earliest grippers were unmarked, opportunities for misidentification and the resulting misstatements were bountiful. While it wasn't IronMind's intention to feed this trend, our Silver Crush Grippers were also sold without any permanent markings. Thus if someone, for example, closed a gripper that was a No. 2 but was told—or wanted to believe—it was a No. 3, that is just what it came to be whenever the story of his conquest was repeated.

We have heard stories going back to the early 1990s of people referring to any really tough gripper they had as a "No. 3," even if in fact it not only wasn't a No. 3, but also wasn't even an IronMind gripper: that this was happening is further testimony to how well-known our grippers had already become. The power of our trademark is also noteworthy since even when people don't use the full product name, i.e. IronMind No. 3 Captains of Crush Gripper, whether they shorten it to IronMind #3, CoC3, No. 3, or even just 3, it is fully recognized as one of IronMind's grippers. Needless to say, whenever we hear about a misidentification or false claim about our grippers, we try to set the record straight. If you ever have a comment or a question about our grippers, please feel free to contact us directly—we're here to help you out.

Growing up

Early evolution and the birth of the Trainer

In late 1992, as part of our march toward the elusive perfect product, IronMind brought all design and manufacturing elements of our grippers in-house, freeing Warren Tetting to continue to make grippers in his signature style, while allowing IronMind to move forward with our ideas about how to continue the evolution of our grippers according to our vision of improved precision, durability, and appearance. Recognizing that most people could not close our No. 1 gripper right out of the box and that the gap between a typical sporting goods store gripper and our No. 1 was too large for most people to bridge, we acted on a suggestion from Major Al Bunting, and our Trainer was born. Far from being a wimpy gripper, the Trainer (c. 100 lb.) is where most people begin their journey up the grip mountain. By its very character and construction, it is leagues apart from a mass-market gripper, and when you give it a try, you will see that compared to traditional grippers, closing a Trainer is nothing to sneeze at.

The next generation of Silver Crush Grippers, which IronMind began selling in 1993, incorporated a number of design advances, and they were easily recognized by the stainless steel handles we introduced into the gripper world that year, and by the clear band at the midpoint of the knurled handle, which has been a signature element in our trade dress ever since. Interestingly, one of the first copycat products initially mimicked even this detail—kind of like the rip-off jeans that copied Levi's signature red tab label. If you can't innovate, you imitate, and when IronMind politely requested that the manufacturer stop infringing our mark, he proved his creativity by replacing the one band . . . with two!

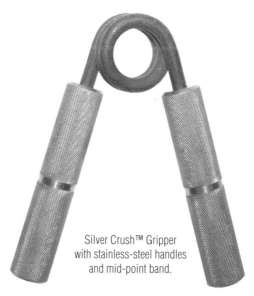

Silver Crush™ Gripper with stainless-steel handles and mid-point band.

IronMind also pioneered a new assembly technique that freed our grippers from the key disadvantages associated with the traditional drift pin method (used to hold the spring in the handles) previously developed by Warren Tetting. Do not construe this as criticism of Warren's drift pin technique, as it has certain advantages too, but IronMind developed an alternative approach that gave us a set of trade-off values we preferred. Incidentally, it's quite an exclusive club of people who own a very rare, limited-production gripper we made in this era: it had stainless steel handles and used a right-hand wind spring, a product configuration that had a short life span, in part because our customers didn't like it compared to our traditional left-hand wind springs. And if you didn't know that springs could be right- or left-handed, we'll touch more on that later.

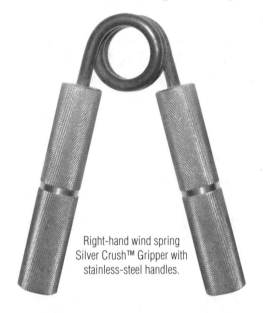

Right-hand wind spring Silver Crush™ Gripper with stainless-steel handles.

By now we had already made significant progress in improving some of the key functions of IronMind grippers—with big gains in accuracy, durability and appearance—but little did we know how much more progress we would make in the coming years. Specifically, we took a number of steps to continue increasing both the consistency and the life span of our grippers, but there is something else we did in 1993 that forevermore changed the gripper market: we began stamping our trademark (T, 1, 2, 3, 4) on the ends of the handles. Now there was no more possibility of confusing what you or your buddy had closed, and these trademarks, even in their simplest and most incomplete forms, are some of the most well-recognized product names in the entire strength world. In later years, we added five new models: first, the Guide (G) and the Sport (S) in 2004, and then the Nos. 1.5, 2.5, and 3.5 in 2006.

By the way, the issue of life span seldom comes up in discussions of Captains of Crush Grippers because so few of the people who talk the most about IronMind's early grippers have any direct experience with how quickly they broke compared to the grippers IronMind makes today. In fact, increased durability was one of the first areas where we made a quantum leap forward when we brought the manufacturing of IronMind grippers in-house. We have continued on this path, and over the years, we have succeeded in substantially boosting the life span of our grippers. This isn't important just in terms of having your favorite gripper around for a good long while: as we'll see later, this fact figures prominently into understanding some commonly repeated misstatements about our Silver Crush Grippers.

March toward perfection
One of the reasons why Captains of Crush Grippers are the leader is because IronMind has been serious about making grippers that give better training results. Sure, good-looking grippers are nice and tough grippers are nice, but we also wanted to develop training tools for serious strength athletes, and this was no easy target. We think that IronMind has some of the world's most demanding users, and to meet their needs, we try to tap our immersion in the strength world to gain a unique perspective. We pair that knowledge and our willingness to chart new territory with the goal of designing the equipment that produces the best training results. Take something as simple as the handle on a gripper.

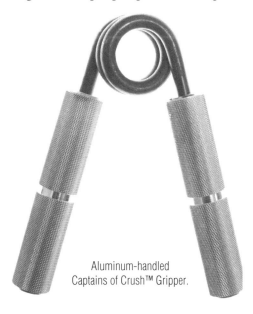
Aluminum-handled Captains of Crush™ Gripper.

After trying several types of steel handles and finishes on our grippers over our first few years of production, in 1995 we changed to aluminum—a revolutionary move at the time, and another example of how Captains of Crush Grippers have set the pace in product features and product quality. We felt that aluminum, while expensive, was functionally superior to steel for our application in a number of key ways, not the least of which was the way it knurled and the way it felt in your hand compared to our steel-handled grippers. Anyone who has tried one of our Silver Crush Grippers can vouch for how the chrome-plated handle always had a slick feeling, even in a well-chalked hand, and how especially if you were doing repetitions, it was hard to keep the gripper in its sweet spot without frequently repositioning it in your hand as it squirmed around. When we introduced aluminum handles, they raised some eyebrows, so we held our breath. Fortunately this giant step forward was accepted by the market.

It used to be that cheap imported grippers were easy to spot—they had telltale plastic handles and light, little springs. A few years ago, though, showing the global impact of Captains of Crush Grippers, cheap imports started showing up with aluminum handles and thicker springs. With a wholesale price of a couple of dollars, you shouldn't expect perfection, and that's why these grippers, for example, are a little crude, vary from batch to batch, and get easier the more you squeeze them.

Meanwhile, Captains of Crush Grippers, while cosing a few dollars more, continue to be made in the USA, and as the gold standard in the grip world, they offer the kind of quality that you deserve if you are serious about your training.

The pond grows

Bob Bollenbach's gym
Richard Sorin undoubtedly provided the original inspiration for many people to develop and demonstrate world-class hand strength by closing a No. 3 Captains of Crush Gripper, but things had progressed a lot since those earliest days, and in our thinking it was a guy named Ron Mazza who marked the beginning of the next generation of grip men—guys who pushed standards up to a new level. Ron came from Bollenbach's Gym, and longtime IronMind customers know that Bob Bollenbach was a grip maniac. Bob, as I, was charmed by an old Iron Man gripper, and in a time-honored tradition he had one hanging in the gas station where he worked, along with the

standing offer that if you closed the gripper, you'd get a free tank of gas. Bob never gave away any free gas, but when IronMind started selling grippers, he quickly heard about what we were doing, and suffice it to say that with this introduction in 1991, Bob Bollenbach had very special status at IronMind. Bob used to pick through his orders back then and was known to send back some of the grippers because he felt they weren't up to snuff (Bob set the bar very high, so we knew that if he liked a gripper, it had to be good).

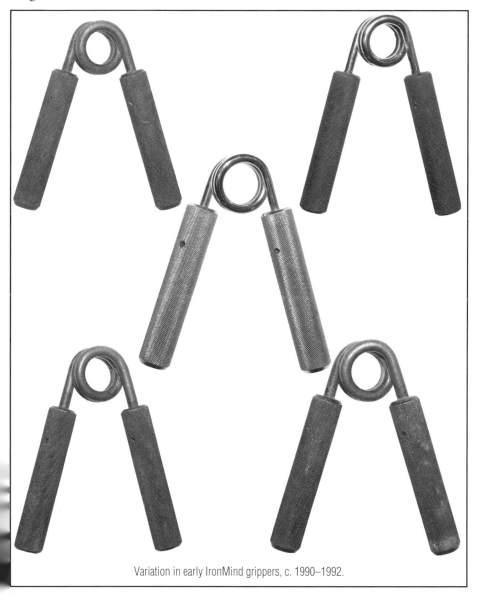

Variation in early IronMind grippers, c. 1990–1992.

We should digress a little at this point to explain that because of the manufacturing variations of those grippers from the very early 1990s, especially before IronMind brought its manufacturing in-house, we could comb through our inventory and find some grippers that were wider, some that were narrower, some that had a more deeply-set spring, and some that had a larger gap between the bottom of the spring coil and the top of the handles, and so forth—all of which made picking an order for Bob Bollenbach something like selecting the mushrooms for a gourmet chef. We always held our breath and lived in fear of what Bob would say when he got his order: "Well, Randy, I liked most of the grippers, but I am sending one back." Later, as our grippers evolved, Bob stopped returning grippers to us, which we took as an indication of the progress we had made from the old days.

Incidentally, talking about being able to hand pick grippers with certain characteristics back in the early 1990s, the following example emphasizes how much things have changed with IronMind grippers since those earliest days, underlining the advances we have been able to make in the consistency and precision of Captain of Crush Grippers.

A few years ago, we got a request from a guy who asked if we could find him an easier No. 3. We wrote back explaining that while we might have been able to do that in 1990, those days were long gone and now this would be kind of like trying to find him a light 20-kg Eleiko IWF-certified barbell plate. We went on to explain that our latest grippers have always been our best grippers because over the years IronMind has continued to refine and improve its product. This piece of information resulted in an Internet post about how we had established a "new" standard for our grippers, and from that, myths about our latest grippers experienced a viral growth spurt before expiring. Now when someone asks about getting a gripper that might be narrower or wider, easier or harder, than his last one, we usually explain that this is not possible as we aim for the bull's eye with each Captains of Crush Gripper.

Ron Mazza

It was fitting that Ron Mazza came from Bob Bollenbach's gym because this gave Ron a chance to run through Bob's substantial gripper collection, which established something of a yardstick for comparing Ron's performances to earlier standards. Over the years, Bob had been known to press his grippers on everyone from Bill Kazmaier to Richard Sorin, and Bob described Ron's capabilities against other people he had seen perform on them by saying, "There is no comparison," so that should tell you something about Ron's grip strength. Ron Mazza's role in the history of Captains of Crush Grippers is also significant for a reason that I have explained over the years but has largely gone unnoticed, even though it is very illuminating when the discussion turns to IronMind's "old" grippers versus our "new" grippers.

Ron's certification came after IronMind had advanced from our earliest grippers—he was the first person who made the grade after IronMind's earliest grippers had been replaced with improved versions. This is important because it should dispel the haughty and misguided claim that the guys who were certified after the earliest grippers were discontinued somehow didn't really measure up to the very first guys IronMind certified. In actuality, we believe that one of IronMind's responsibilities is to ensure that we preserve the legacy of these unique grippers, and we do this by keeping an eye firmly fixed on the historical record. To do this, we complement our internal resources with input from key members of the worldwide grip community as part of IronMind's system for quality control and for maintaining checks and balances. We ask key customers, "What do you think?" trying to learn from their comments.

Rising standards

We sometimes shake our heads in amazement when we hear the related comment that we must be making our grippers easier and easier since more and more guys have been certified on the No. 3. Here's part of the answer.

Students of modern grip history know that Richard Sorin discovered and named the Blob (it's the sawed-off end from a cast York 100-lb. dumbbell) and that even when he stood alone as being certified on our No. 3, Richard considered lifting the Blob to be his most meritorious feat of grip strength, something he said he could only do some of the time, and then it was usually a full deadlift at best ("This is probably the toughest grip feat I have ever done," Richard said).

In stark contrast, now there are guys who can clean it, pass it around their bodies, and even snatch it. Are Blobs getting lighter? Is the York Barbell Company part of some greater conspiracy to sweep earlier grip masters off their exclusive perches? Of course not. How about this screamingly obvious explanation instead: with more strong guys trying to lift Blobs, the standards are rising, just as they do in any sport as it matures. It's really just that simple.

On the other hand, a little later we'll tell you the rest of the story, as the late Paul Harvey would say, because we do want to say more about the world famous No. 3 and because there are some points about certification on it (and the No. 3.5 and the No. 4) that should see the light of day.

Enter the No. 4—and Joe Kinney

Recognizing what was coming—that grip standards were on the rise—even though the No. 3 CoC was the universally recognized mark of a world-class grip, we knew that we had guys prowling the earth who could do more, so we created the No. 4 Captains of Crush Gripper in 1994.

When IronMind developed the No. 4, our idea was that it would represent the newly established uppermost echelon in our family of Captains of Crush Grippers, one that might not be reached for years, but one that would mark the strength of guys who were head and shoulders above even a mighty No. 3 Captains of Crush Gripper. When it was originally introduced, we would often tell people who wanted to buy it that they could save their money and simply squeeze a brick, because that's about what squeezing a No. 4 Captains of Crush Gripper felt like. Also, we would explain that if you had someone who could do, say, 10 or 12 full, consecutive reps on a No. 1—not world-class but definitely a person with well above average grip strength—you would have to look closely to see that he had even moved the No. 4 when he gave it his best effort.

We went over three years before it was closed officially, but even before he finally succeeded as the first to reach this milestone, Joe Kinney was dogging the No. 4 CoC with a level of determination and fight that we had never before seen in the grip world.

Most people do not realize just how prodigiously gifted Richard Sorin was: he used to tell me that he never really trained his grip in a systematic way, but just performed spontaneously. This was a guy, you have to remember, who told me he could pinch grip a pair of 35s when he was 12 years old.

Joe Kinney was cut from a different cloth, however—a guy with a past marked by health problems, but who wouldn't take no for an answer. When Joe Kinney first called to order a gripper, I talked him into ordering a No. 2 instead of the No. 3 Joe wanted to buy. Shortly after, Joe got bored with his No. 2, got the No. 3 he'd wanted in the first place, closed it, and then—hold onto your hat—he became the first—and for a long time, the only—person in the world to close the No. 4.

Joe first stalked the No. 4 with the single-mindedness of a hungry predator and then closed in for the kill with the same unwavering focus, and in the process, he didn't just raise the bar, he advanced grip training. Joe developed innovative training strategies for grip work, and through a combination of increased volume and intensity, set a new high-water mark in the field. Joe also set himself apart by neither walking around endlessly beating his chest nor idly chatting nor slinging buckets of mud at others; he just quietly took care of business, and before he was done, he gave the grip world quite a jolt.

Potatoes vs. soda cans
I have told this story to a few people over the years, but it is worth repeating here.

Years ago, when they alone ruled the pinnacle of the grip world, I asked Richard Sorin and John Brookfield what they each thought about someone being able to crush a potato and burst a can of beer or soda. Richard said he thought the can was possible, but the potato was humanly impossible; John said he thought the potato was possible, but the can wasn't (John, very much to his credit, would later say that he was wrong about the can and became very proficient at bursting cans himself).

The first point is that the two top grip guys at that time were in striking disagreement, but the second point is the one that is really telling: along came Joe Kinney and he could do both things. Joe Kinney was the first person IronMind certified for closing our No. 4 Captains of Crush Gripper, and he was also the first person who ever sent us any proof that he could close a No. 3 with only two fingers—something that used to make people dizzy when they just considered the possibility of this being done.

Later in this book (see Chapter 6), you will have a chance, in Joe's words, to learn how he trained. "In Joe's words" is vital here because there is at least one highly-hyped e-book on the market that supposedly presents Kinney's training adapted, when in actuality, its biggest contribution is to teach guys who can't close a gripper over its full, natural range how to deep-set it for a partial movement. If you think this e-book really portrays how Joe Kinney trained, just compare its advice to what Joe has written later in this book, or if you ever have a chance to meet Joe in person, ask him how well he knows the author of this e-book and what he thinks of its accuracy.

Incidentally, making history—even relatively obscure grip history—isn't without its risks, as success can arouse envy and jealousy in others. For example, a particularly strident critic of Joe Kinney once sent me a two-page e-mail describing why and how it was physically impossible to burst a beer can, using this shaky platform as part of the basis for his assault on Joe. By now, any number of guys probably would be happy to prove that they, too, can burst beer cans, as it's now a quite well-established feat of strength.

Holles of fame
MILO readers have been introduced to a special family in Wales (UK) where having incredible grip strength seems to fit hand in glove with equally unusual levels of modesty and a zeal for doing things properly. I am referring to the Holle family, of which five of the brothers—Nathan, Gavin, Craig, Jay and Kayne—have been certified as closing the No. 3 Captains of Crush Gripper, and Nathan has been certified as closing the No. 4, the second man in history to accomplish this tremendous feat of grip strength. As I have often written, I cannot say enough good things about these guys—

they quietly do the job in a most remarkable way, and while others are talking, the Holles are training and gaining.

Shortly after Nathan Holle was certified on the No. 4, I received a letter saying what a stir this had created because a group of people didn't believe that Nathan's training could be as straightforward as what he had described. He must be holding something back, or worse, is what I was told was being said on the Internet. His training routine is just too simple, the critics charged.

We have long observed that some of the people who are most outspoken yet off-base about both IronMind grippers and grip training in general have relatively little experience in the larger lifting or strength world, creating knowledge gaps when it comes to grip-specific stuff. As a quick test of my hypothesis, I asked someone who has never been to a world weightlifting championships or an Olympic Games, but who has read *MILO* diligently from the very first issue, the following question:

"If I told you that someone said Nathan's training is too simple to work—quick!—what would you say?"

"The Bulgarians . . ."

"Right," I said. "You just got an A+ on the test."

The Bulgarians, of course, are some of the most feared weightlifters on the face of the earth and they have a tradition of notching their belts with triple(!) bodyweight clean and jerks. You read that right: triple bodyweight clean and jerks. And the hallmark of how these guys train is not some mind-numbing combination of this, that and the other, or some other mumbo jumbo they got from an online Wizard of Odd. They snatch, clean and jerk, and squat. With really heavy weights. Over and over again. And they get world-record strong.

Remember this story when you read Nathan Holle's section (see Chapter 7) about training on Captains of Crush Grippers.

Five more make ten: a growing family

Starting off easy
In response to requests for a Captains of Crush Gripper that covered the territory between the traditional plastic-handled sporting goods store gripper (which generally runs in the range of 30 to 50 lb. of resistance) and our Trainer Captains of Crush Gripper rated at 100 lb., IronMind added two new grippers to the CoC family in 2004. The Guide, c. 60 lb., defined the high-end of the strength levels of sporting goods store grippers—but with the solid construction, precision, and durability of all our Captains of Crush Grippers. The Sport, c. 80 lb. of resistance, was a stepping stone to the Trainer and a way to condition the hands and to warm up.

Filling in the gaps
Periodically, IronMind would receive requests for grippers halfway between our benchmark grippers, for example, between the No. 2 and the No. 3. For years we resisted, in part because the traditional steps in our gripper line had been in place and had worked for years, and in part because we knew of manufacturers who had tried to do this and the grippers they produced tended to overlap from one category to another. Another factor was that over the years, IronMind had produced a steady stream of grip-training tools so that today's aspiring grip master could go into battle with plenty of choices in armaments besides just grippers. Still, we could understand the appeal of this concept and in 2006, we determined that we could effectively split the ranges in between our well-established grippers in a way that satisfied our quality-control standards. IronMind launched three new models within the Captains of Crush family: the No. 1.5, the No. 2.5, and the No. 3.5. And just as their names implied, these grippers represented the half steps between the No. 1 and the No. 2, the No. 2 and the No. 3, and the No. 3 and the No. 4, respectively.

As ever, though, there is a difference between what works in theory and in tests and what performs as predicted in the field, so we waited to see how the results would fall.

Interestingly, one of the best indications that we'd hit our mark came from a customer who called to say that he couldn't feel any difference between his

No. 1 and his No. 1.5 gripper, and he was concerned that perhaps we had made a mistake. Within minutes, though, we found out that he could do about a dozen reps on his No. 1, but only a few on his No. 1.5. "That's the difference," we said. After a pause, mulling it over, he said, "Yeah, now I get it. Thanks much, that's perfect."

It's like a 10-lb. plate and a 5-kg (11-lb.) plate . . . grab one and then the other and you're unlikely to say that you can feel a difference—after all, we're only talking about a 1 lb. difference. But if you pile 10-lb. plates on one bar and the same number of 5-kg plates on another and go to failure on both, the difference will be apparent.

And from the guys who could certify on the No. 3 and were eyeing the No. 4, we also got the correct pattern. The ones who could just barely close the No. 3 still had air between the handles on the No. 3.5, while the ones who could dominate the No. 3 and were drawing nearer to the No. 4 could fully close the No. 3.5, even if they weren't quite there yet on the No. 4.

Finally, how did our bridge grippers stack up as training tools? After all, we developed these grippers with the idea that they would help guys make progress, moving up a level or two in the Captains of Crush chain. If you want to be tough about it, all those things described so far are nice, but in the end, IronMind designs and builds Captains of Crush Grippers for training—we want results we can see. Testimonials started flowing in: "Thank you for the No. 1.5; now I know I will be able to close a CoC 2" . . . "The #2.5 is just what I need. I hope to get certified on the 3 later this year." Again and again we would see and hear about how the latest Captains of Crush Grippers were doing their job—increasing grip strength—and the reason why is very simple: lower reps are better than higher reps for building maximum strength, and with more levels of Captains of Crush Grippers to choose from, it was easier for people to train in the optimum rep range for increasing strength.

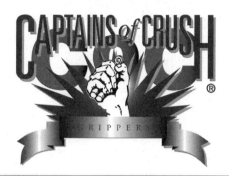

Chapter 2
Understanding Calibration: A Technical Twist

Calibration and what it means

Based on our research and our sales experience, the earliest grippers IronMind sold, while certainly more variable than what we sell today, were by no means as inconsistent as a few detractors claimed. Because of our familiarity with the tolerances of the sacred coin of our realm—barbell plates—we introduced the analogy of uncalibrated barbell plates to explain the precision level of our grippers.

How precise is that puppy?
Most people who lift weights probably don't know that the average barbell plate has an accuracy level in the range of 5–10%, and that accuracy levels of 2–3% are considered very good (and that sort of tolerance just happens to coincide very nicely with some of the general limits of what humans can detect as a noticeable difference). In other words, that uncalibrated plate that says 45 lb. on it will probably weigh somewhere between about 40 and 50 lb., or maybe somewhere between 43 and 47, and it might even fall

within a narrower range, but it is extremely unlikely to be exactly 45 lb. That's the nature of an uncalibrated barbell plate.

An International Weightlifting Federation (IWF)-certified calibrated plate, on the other hand, is so hair-splittingly precise that you can use one to check the accuracy of a scale, which is part of the reason why, in 2009, an IWF-certified 20-kg Eleiko bumper plate, for example, costs over $300 in the U.S. (yes, that is correct, over $300 for one plate, without shipping).

How precise are these plates? Hold three U.S. quarters or three one-euro coins in your hand: the three quarters will give you an approximate idea of the maximum amount a 20-kg plate can be overweight and still get an IWF certification, while the three euros would cause the plate to flunk. And if you think that's less of a difference than you could possibly notice when you're lifting, you are correct, and consider that the amount a plate can be underweight and still get certified is half of how much it can be overweight!

Calibration: what it is and isn't
Unfortunately, from here, if you didn't know all of this about competitive lifting nor understand how barbell plates are calibrated, you might mistakenly think you could calibrate a gripper. And in fact, that is just what happened: people in the grip community thought that by simply testing a gripper and noting its resistance that it was "calibrated." Of course, if that were true, the same process would make all barbell plates calibrated just by weighing them—a fundamental misunderstanding of the idea of calibration. Even more extreme, if this were true, then a manhole cover would be "calibrated" just by weighing it precisely. We will have more on this boondoggle a little later in this book (see Chapter 3).

The truth is that barbell plates can be and are calibrated for specific reasons, using processes that do not apply as directly to grippers, and there are lessons to be learned from both the correct and incorrect use of this term.

First, in actuality, calibration is not a matter of taking a static snapshot of something and reporting on what you find, but rather it is a matter of ensuring that something conforms to pre-established criteria, such as the rigid guidelines for competition bumper plates established by the IWF.

Think about beginning with a nearly-perfect but just barely overweight bumper plate, for example, and then removing minute amounts of material from designated portions of the plate until it is within the narrow tolerances allowed by the IWF—and when it finally matches those specifications, it is, in fact, calibrated. Also, please understand that its weight is not the only quality that has to meet a specified standard in order for a plate to be calibrated—and that the plates are not the only elements of the certified barbell that are approved for the highest levels of competition.

On the other hand, even though the concept of calibration has a history of being misunderstood and abused in the gripper world, the worst offenders have contributed something of value, even if unwittingly. Why? Because regardless of the term's misuse, talk of calibration increased awareness of such topics as consistency in grippers, and along with the negative baggage, some good things followed. We, at least, redoubled our efforts to understand and control the factors that influenced a gripper's performance in order to increase the consistency of Captains of Crush Grippers.

Grippers: no magic numbers
Even more crucial than grasping what calibration actually means in the lifting world, though, is the fundamental fact that grippers, unlike barbell plates, do not automatically lend themselves to an indisputable magic number as a measure of their difficulty. This concept isn't intuitively obvious but it is central to understanding gripper ratings and related topics.

What does this mean?

To begin with, if I tell you that something is a 25-lb. barbell plate or 50-kg barbell plate, for example, you have a sense of what that really means, both relatively and absolutely. In other words, if you lift weights, you know about what it feels like to lift a 25-lb. plate and about what it feels like compared to a 50-kg plate. Why?

It's because the force required to overcome a barbell plate once it's loaded on a standard bar is simply a function of its mass (or weight), so all you have to do is plunk it on a precise scale, read the number, and—*voilà*—that's a true index of what we can call its degree of difficulty: unflinchingly, barbell plates with more mass (e.g., the 50-kg plate) are heavier and are more difficult to lift than barbell plates that have less mass (e.g., the 25-lb. plate).

A gripper using a torsion spring fitted with handles is an entirely different animal, one which involves in a dramatic way such factors as hand position and the surface of the handles—this is before even beginning to talk about the spring involved. Thus, even if you begin with an absolutely precise spring, sliding your hand up and down the handles of any gripper changes the amount of force required to close it. In that sense, any gripper of this type could be called adjustable, since one's leverage changes depending upon one's position on the handles.

Similarly, whether or not a given gripper is stabilized when squeezed, has good knurling, is squeezed with a dry hand or an oily one, and so forth, will make a dramatic difference in your ability to close it, even when the spring in all these instances is precisely the same. Incidentally, specific training techniques based on these principles have been developed over the years, which certainly validate how factors other than spring-specific characteristics affect how difficult a particular gripper is to close: use of chalk, finger placement on the handle, and careful positioning of the gripper, for example, can give you a definite edge when closing it.

Continuing with the comparison between a gripper and a barbell plate, take four IWF-certified 25-kg plates and put two on an IWF-certified bar and put the other two on a smooth, dead-stiff, non-revolving, two-inch thick bar; and then do a power clean with each barbell. Notice any difference in difficulty? "Of course," you say. "The first lift is easy and the other one is a lot harder." That's the kind of situation you are dealing with when it comes to a hand gripper. Even if you start off with absolutely identical springs, the other components of the gripper can make a significant difference in how difficult it is to close. It gets trickier still, though, because springs like this can never be as blindingly precise as calibrated plates.

Spring variations
Springs themselves, the units that provide the resistance in grippers, are a formed part, so variations from piece to piece are to be expected. How big

the variations are, however, depends on everything from the inherent limitations of the design to the specifics used in manufacturing and assembling the particular parts. Without getting too wonkish about this, let's roll up our sleeves and take a quick look at how grippers work, and then start to put together all of these pieces to assess just how accurate Captains of Crush Grippers really are.

The basic technical things to understand about torsion springs are that their strength will be a function of a number of factors (such as the wire diameter used, the diameter and the number of coils, the angle of the arms, and so forth) and that variations in these parameters and in the final assembly will lead to variations in the load required to deflect the spring. As you can imagine, this situation presents manifold opportunities for differences in what is supposed to be an essentially uniform product, and as you can guess, it's cheaper and easier to make mediocre springs than it is to make really good ones.

The quality level of grippers varies from manufacturer to manufacturer, and certainly some grippers are mere toys and some are fairly junky, but it also is possible to make competition-grade grippers of outstanding quality . . . we feel that Captains of Crush Grippers stand as the living proof. This was no easy thing to achieve, though—we know how much research, thought, time, money and effort it has taken to bring Captains of Crush Grippers to their current levels of sophistication, and they're still not as precise as a calibrated Eleiko barbell plate! Still, by the time we hit our eighth generation of springs, we could see that we had covered a lot of territory since starting in this business. Proprietary IronMind GR8™ springs aren't just a pretty face: they're accurate and tough, too.

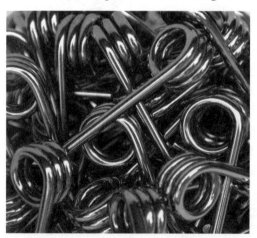
GR8™ Springs—our eighth generation—are available only on CoCs and IMTUGs.

IronMind has long marched to the drum of product quality, and our leadership in making precise grippers reflects our orientation.

Tolerances: how much do they vary?
Since 1990, IronMind has worked steadily to understand and control the factors that might cause variations in how difficult a gripper is to close, and anyone who has a sample of our grippers from, say, 1990 and compares them to a sample from, say, 2008 can confirm that we have been able to make remarkable progress over the years, so much so that we have reached unprecedented levels of consistency and precision. The grippers we sold in 1990 are the ones that varied the most, and they are also the ones that were not made in-house, but frankly, we always liked them and still think they were pretty good. The grippers we make today have an accuracy level that has never before been achieved with a product of this type and amazes both independent reviewers and our hardcore users even if there's still room for improvement. "Enough theory," you say, "what's the bottom line? How much do grippers really vary and what level of difference really makes a difference?" Good questions.

Even the earliest grippers we sold were within the accuracy range of standard (uncalibrated) barbell plates, and our grippers now are pushing the envelope to the point where they are probably more accurate than most of the barbell plates you lift. Returning to those grippers from the early 1990s, they had, for example, variations in the angles in the range of plus or minus about two or three degrees and variations in load of about 10%. As noted earlier, this sort of variation is still within industry standards for springs of this type, and a lot of grippers aren't close to being this accurate.

Incidentally, in 1998 Richard Sorin expressed concern that his "new" gripper was much easier to close than his "old" gripper, and he sent us his test results to demonstrate his point.

Remembering that Richard's true original gripper would have actually been an Iron Man gripper, not an IronMind gripper, it is still instructive to look at Richard's results since they probably present a worst-case scenario, given that Richard's point was that his "old" gripper was much tougher to close than his "new" one. Using a weight stack and noting "all grippers tested and re-tested—same results—all in same steady vertical position," Richard reported to us, with an illustration of both his testing procedure and the results, that it took an additional 20 lb. of pressure to close his "old" gripper than his "new" gripper.

These results, indeed, both confirm that his older gripper was tougher than the newer one, as Richard had said, and that this issue had been exaggerated and distorted by some people since the size of the difference was consistent with exactly what we had been saying for years: it was within the range typical of all the barbell plates likely to be found in any gym. It's no coincidence that about this time, a customer sent us a list of the 45-lb. plates he had weighed in his gym and was more than mildly surprised to find that while some were heavier, some were lighter than their face value. This is the typical variation we mentioned earlier, something that isn't known by everyone who lifts weights, even if it's old hat to people involved with weightlifting at the World Championships or Olympics level, for example, or to the guys like Steve Justa who lift huge piles of junk but who actually weigh what they lift.

Still, as much as we admire and strive for top quality at IronMind, we are the first to tell people that if all they have to train with is the world's most imprecise gripper, not to worry about it and just train their guts out anyway, because it's how hard and smart you train, not how fancy your equipment is, that's most important to your progress. Later, when you can afford it, you can move up to better equipment, and the good news here is that buying a world-class gripper is only a few dollars more than something inferior.

Misperceptions of variability
From time to time, we hear someone say, "I was over at my buddy's house last night and his No. 1 gripper seemed so much tougher/easier than mine." When someone calls IronMind to ask about a Captains of Crush Gripper that they think is out of spec, the first question we ask is, "Do you lift weights?" Why? Because the frame of reference of a lifter with some experience is vastly different from a non-lifter when it comes to maximum performances.

Suppose that you've been lifting weights for a while and that your best deadlift is 500 lb. What happens when you load up your PR deadlift and try it at different gyms (or with different plates in the same gym) or at different times? Everyone who has lifted for a while understands that sometimes 500 lb. feels like a feather and at other times it feels like a ton. Your experience has taught you that as much as you might like to, you will not be able to duplicate this maximum lift at all times and in all places—and because it's your max, you can't lift even 1 lb. more. The same thing applies to your maximum performance on a gripper. And unless the conditions under which you attempt a maximum effort are similar on the critical dimensions, direct comparisons from one effort to the next are invalid.

If you just barely closed a No. 2 Captains of Crush Gripper when you were fresh, properly warmed-up, and had a pile of your best buddies cheering you on, you would expect to perform at a lower level when you were tired and picked up the gripper cold and your social context was a goldfish, right? Nonetheless, especially among non-lifters, somewhat different performances under conditions as variable as these leads them to conclude that their gripper was faulty.

When a person calls and says that he just got a Captains of Crush Gripper that was significantly different from his friend's and something must be wrong with it, we start by asking a few questions. We might learn that he closed his friend's gripper under the first set of conditions and then a week later, he got a new gripper of his own and, under the second set of conditions, he missed closing it by "the thickness of a sheet of paper." By the end of the conversation, all parties are in agreement that the two Captains of Crush Grippers sound like identical twins and—*voila!*—a few days later, the person is closing the gripper that he had first thought was "vastly harder."

In a related error, we have had people sound the alarm because when they measured their gripper through its packaging, they thought the handle spread was off by .002". Yet, in the same breath, the width of a credit card might mistakenly be reported as 2-1/4" when, in fact, it's 2-1/8". Anyone with reasonable eyesight and even a child's ruler should be able to measure the width of a credit card accurately; and a professional machinist, trained to measure things very precisely, would probably writhe at the idea of measuring a gripper to a thousandth of an inch through its packaging and would be the first to use a word like "about" when reporting a measurement obtained this way.

The moral of this story is that while it's certainly true that there are plenty of grippers on the market that do vary all over the board, they are not Captains of Crush Grippers. Captains of Crush Grippers, as we have long said, are far more accurate than the barbell plates you are probably training with, so if you are looking for explanations of performance difference, first look at the size of the difference and then consider the circumstances.

Getting a Handle on the Numbers

To be honest about it, we sometimes hear gripper stories—tales of phantom grippers, outstanding performances by mythical characters, and numbers or measurements—that make us cringe. Fortunately, at least some of the time, we can take such conversation from the level of fuzzy and speculative to precise and objective, as in the following example:

Another Gripper Myth Bites the Dust

IronMind got an e-mail from a customer who is something of a gripper fanatic—he said that a No. 3 Captains of Crush Gripper that he'd recently purchased had "uneven handles . . .," explaining that "one handle is placed higher than the other."

This customer said that the handles were not just slightly off, but so far off that he felt the gripper was defective and dysfunctional (incidentally, it's probably relevant to point out that it's a challenge gripper that he can't yet fully close).

Knowing that anything is possible, IronMind was quick to acknowledge what he said and suggested that one handle might well be 1 or 2 mm below the other, in which case we would consider this more cosmetic than func-

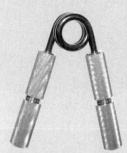

tional, also noting that if it were 5 or 10 mm off, we would consider the gripper to be defective.

The customer was perfectly clear: "It's definitely not 1 or 2 mm . . . I didn't measure it but I would say probably 1/2" or 12 mm."

Well, when IronMind received the gripper, we did measure it, extremely precisely, and the gap was . . . 2 mm.

This gripper has a 2-mm gap that a customer reported as 12 mm.

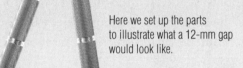

Here we set up the parts to illustrate what a 12-mm gap would look like.

Reprinted from the IronMind News, July 16, 2009:
http://www.ironmind.com/ironmind/opencms/Articles/2009/Jul/Another_Gripper_Myth_Bites_the_Dust.html

As you can see in the photo, there is a big difference even visually between a handle that is off 2 mm and one that is off 12 mm. Suffice it to say, it's important to keep small differences in perspective and focus not on scrutinizing your gripper but on training with it.

Accurate and longer lasting, too
Even though we hold our earliest IronMind grippers in high regard, we have come a long way from those days, which is reflected in the comments we get from people applauding the consistency of the latest Captains of Crush Grippers. Today's Captains of Crush Grippers have set new standards for precision, appearance, and longevity. This last point is a significant one that is highly appreciated by anyone who might have owned one of our Silver Crush Grippers from the early 1990s: they had a fraction of the life span of our latest Captains of Crush Grippers, and the difference is so significant that we can best illustrate it by noting that anyone who shows you an old Silver Crush Gripper that is still in one piece is also showing you

a gripper that wasn't closed too many times—if it had been, it would have broken!

How about the easy ones?!
Stories abound about some ferociously hard gripper that so-and-so supposedly closed, and it certainly is true that the grippers we sold in the early 1990s varied more widely than those we sell today. This means that it is true that some were unusually tough, but it is also true that some were unusually easy, so don't ever be conned into thinking that all those really "old" grippers were especially hard. Also, always remember the quick test regarding our Silver Crush Grippers: if it's still in one piece, it simply was never closed too many times. Further, because the easier Silver Crush Grippers were closed the most and therefore broke the most, this means that the easiest ones are long gone, while only the hardest ones remain, and this simple fact has distorted ideas about how tough they were to close.

Now that you know more about their family history and characteristics, you can keep tales about Silver Crush Grippers in their proper perspective and, given their limited life span, if you're a collector, you'll also want to keep your Silver Crush Grippers reserved for special occasions. Finally, as ever, if you're stumped about gripper variation, you are always welcome to contact IronMind and we will be happy to try to get to the bottom of the mystery.

Phantom 4s and other mythological creatures
In 1992 Warren Tetting made three grippers for IronMind that had springs that were slightly thicker than those we had been using in our No. 3 grippers. Of course, we sent one to Richard Sorin and one to John Brookfield, and even though we never received any corroboration for it, Richard told us that he closed it and we believe him. Nonetheless, the idea that this gripper is a so-called "phantom 4" or "the toughest gripper ever closed" is fiction. Whether you look at the numbers involved in the specific elements of this gripper or just pick it up and squeeze it for yourself, you will accept it for what it is: a gripper that is a little harder than a No. 3, nothing more and nothing less. On the other hand, if we had a dollar for each time we have heard a phantom 4 story or another, Richard and I could go out for a pretty nice dinner.

Calibration – The Short Story

When talking about calibration and grippers, the situation can be summed up by the following points:

1. Calibration means making an object, such as a barbell plate, conform to a pre-defined or already established standard.

2. For example, a calibrated IWF-certified 25-kg bumper plate must match the precise guidelines set forth by the IWF.

3. Throwing a 25-kg barbell plate on a scale and weighing it—however precisely—is not calibrating a barbell plate: it is just weighing a barbell plate.

4. The term calibration is commonly misunderstood and misused in the realm of grippers.

5. Barbell plates lend themselves to calibration more easily than hand grippers. And, unlike weighing a plate on a scale, there is no one universally accepted standard for rating the difficulty of a hand gripper.

6. Thus, rating the strength of a hand gripper is not calibrating a gripper—it is simply measuring the strength of that gripper—using one person's methods, which might differ from another person's.

7. Hand grippers are often assigned strengths based on their perceived difficulty relative to Captains of Crush Grippers. Thus a gripper might be called a 1.13, in that it is felt to be slightly more difficult than an idealized No. 1 Captains of Crush Gripper; or it might be rated as a 3.02, in that it is felt to be a whisper more difficult than an idealized No. 3 CoC Gripper.

8. Captains of Crush Grippers are the established benchmark by which most other hand grippers are measured or compared; thus, while saying something is a "280-lb. gripper" really means very little to most people,

saying that "it feels about like a No. 2 Captains of Crush Gripper" has universal meaning in the strength world.

9. By virtue of having remained true to their deep roots and having reached high levels of precision, and because they are the standard by which other grippers are measured, Captains of Crush Grippers *de facto* can now be called calibrated, in the true sense of the word.

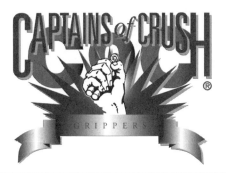

Chapter 3
Poundage Ratings: How Tough Is It to Close?

Testing 1, 2, 3 . . .

In 1993 we began to test grippers, partly to appease Richard Sorin, who kept telling me how I was "really missing the boat" for not describing how much force it took to close the grippers we sold. Richard felt very strongly that it was natural for people to be interested in a quick summary of how hard it was to close a particular gripper, and we could fully appreciate this goal. Testing and rating grippers, however, is not the simple proposition it might appear to be, and the testing process can quickly reveal *naiveté* in everything from lifting in general to grippers specifically; it can also reveal ignorance about even the barest rudiments of how to conduct legitimate research. And, as we'll see, there are even more potential problems if you have a dishonest or biased person conducting the tests.

Time out for testing
To repeat, testing grippers isn't as easy as you might think, and like a chain saw, it will draw blood from an incompetent or unlucky operator in the

blink of an eye—even if operator error might not be quite as obvious to all when it comes to testing grippers.

Consider what would happen if someone launched a testing program that confused different brands of grippers (whether accidentally or intentionally), had a testing method that was neither reliable nor valid (in a formal statistical sense), and selected the worst cases from all the data he had collected and then attributed those to a particular brand of gripper? There was a case like this and even though it occurred about 10 years ago, reviewing it is quite interesting.

The centerpiece of the program was a test that included over 40 grippers, roughly half of which were identified as being IronMind grippers, and the stated purpose of the test was to examine the consistency of the grippers.

Suspect standards
First, we realized that the guy conducting the study had an ulterior motive: he was trying to manufacture and sell an imitation of Captains of Crush Grippers, so his starting point was to denigrate our product, and he would then introduce his copy, which he would tout as vastly superior to the real deal. Since the individual was neither trained in research nor very knowledgeable about grippers, you might wonder why looking at the study had any value, but here's the surprising thing. This report ended up being very useful, so let's take a look at it. In fact, we found that the data it presented clearly demonstrated that what this person claimed about IronMind grippers is false and that what we said about them is true.

Mark Twain once sagely noted, "There are lies, damned lies, and statistics." And the reason why statistics are so often used to mislead the public is because most people have had little chance to learn the basics that will allow them to sort a good number and truthful claim from a bad number and a lie. The statistics that Mark Twain was referring to represent numerical abuse, or simply said, using numbers to mislead by replacing fact with fiction.

The simplest way to understand how numbers can be crunched into statistics is to consider what are called descriptive statistics.

> **Definition**
>
> **Descriptive statistics**
>
> Stastical methods used to summarize or describe a collection of data [in a study]. [These may also include tables and graphs.]
>
> Wikipedia on-line encyclopedia; 8/6/09.

Descriptive statistics, you will be happy to learn, are just what they sound like: think of them as tools that help us to take piles of numbers and describe them in a way that summarizes them accurately and extracts meaning from them. It's like being given a list of how much each person in a group weighs and wanting to describe the typical person's weight based on this overall sample. A statistical measure of what is called central tendency does this job for us and if all of this sounds too heady, you already know exactly what we're talking about: this is what the average is, even if statisticians might be more likely to call it a mean than an average. By either name, it's the same number—calculated the same way and identical in meaning.

> **Definition**
>
> **Measure of central tendency**
>
> An average or number used to represent a group of numbers. The most common type of average is the arithmetic *mean*, which is found by dividing the sum of the scores in the group by the number of members in the group. Other measures include the *median* or middle score, and the *mode*, which is the number occurring most frequently.
>
> The Columbia Electronic Encyclopedia® © 2007, Columbia University Press.

Returning to this report, let's note that in the test, all the grippers in the sample were pooled—that is, the results from the IronMind and non-IronMind grippers were combined—and the worst of the findings were then attributed to IronMind's Captains of Crush Grippers. Hopefully, even a technically unsophisticated reader would notice this egregious error, but for the moment, let's look past it and see how these data allow us to test the claim we have made about IronMind's pattern of progress over the years.

Specifically, let's use these data to assess whether or not IronMind grippers are superior to their competitors and whether IronMind has succeeded in making Captains of Crush Grippers less variable and more consistent over time, marking the sort of evolutionary progress described in Chapter 1.

Reading the tea leaves: a brief lesson in reliability and validity

The research in question used torque ratings as its primary dependent variable for assessing how difficult the grippers were to close—dependent variables are the ones you observe or measure when you are doing an experiment. For example, if you wanted to see if following the *SUPER SQUATS* program made people get bigger and stronger, size and strength (measured before and after someone followed the *SUPER SQUATS* program) would be the dependent variables. For our current purpose, there is no need to focus on either the design of this study or torque ratings *per se* because we knew from field data that we had collected that the torque ratings were neither **reliable** nor **valid**—these are formally defined statistical terms, but they are very easy to understand conceptually.

Reliability
Reliability means that when you repeatedly measure a certain unchanging thing, you should keep getting the same measurement—no room for rubber rulers here. In other words, suppose you keep measuring the length of your kitchen table. If you had an accurate tape measure and knew how to use it, you would get the same measurement each time. If you got a different number each time, that would be a red flag telling you that you had problems with what is called reliability, meaning that the measurements lacked the required level of consistency.

> **Definition**
>
> **Reliability**
>
> Yielding the same or compatible results in different experiments or statistical trials.
>
> *The American Heritage® Dictionary of the English Language, Fourth Edition* ©2000 by Houghton Mifflin Company. Updated in 2003.

Validity

Validity means that the number you get has some relevance to what you are talking about. In this case, torque ratings were presented as the measure of how difficult a gripper was to close, so these torque ratings, if valid, should coincide with perceptions of how tough the grippers felt in your hand. Failure to do that is an indication that the test is invalid, which is a polite way of saying meaningless, and for reasons that we need not go into here, in a very real and quantifiable way, reliability sets an upper limit on validity. In other words, if you start off with an unreliable measure, even if there are no other problems with the design or execution of the research, don't expect it to do very well as far as validity goes.

> **Definition**
>
> **Validity**
>
> The state of being well-grounded or justifiable, being at once relevant and meaningful.
>
> *Merriam-Webster Online Dictionary* © 2009 by Merriam-Webster, Inc.

We knew that when the same grippers were sent back for re-testing, not only the absolute numbers changed, but also the rank orderings. We also knew people who had sent in multiple grippers for testing with this method and this is what happened: the rank ordering of the torque ratings did not correspond with the reality of what the grippers felt like to close (e.g., the gripper with the highest torque rating was not the hardest to close). So much for the torque ratings, as they failed in both reliability and validity, providing numbers that seemed to have the permanence and stability of soap bubbles.

Let's give the other dependent variable, "included angle" (referring to the angle of the spring), the benefit of the doubt and assume it was accurately measured. We would like to march forward and illustrate some things of real value to be gleaned from this report.

Standard deviation: why it's important

Approximately half the grippers in the test were identified as from IronMind, which we will take on faith, and the remainder were reported as coming from other sources, which we will also take on faith. Let's begin, as the author of the report did, and pool the results for each gripper, but instead of stopping here as he did, we will use those numbers as a starting point. Next, we will divide the entire sample into two groups: one includes the grippers identified as coming from IronMind, and the other contains the grippers from other sources. We then further divide the sample, looking at IronMind's Captains of Crush (that is, post-1995) Grippers versus IronMind's pre-Captains of Crush (that is, pre-1995) Grippers. For each of these groups, we calculated the *standard deviation*, which is simply a statistic that measures how much the sample of numbers varies around the mean (average) of the sample. If the numbers vary a lot, the standard deviation goes up, and if they don't vary much, the standard deviation goes down.

> **Definition**
>
> **Standard deviation**
>
> In probability theory and statistics, a measure of the variability or dispersion of a population, a data set, or a probability distribution. A low standard deviation indicates that the data points tend to be very close to the same value (the mean), while a high standard deviation indicates that the data are "spread out" over a large range of values.
>
> Wikipedia on-line encyclopedia; 8/6/09.

For example, if you had one group of three people, all of whom weighed 200 lb., and a second group of three people, where one weighed 100 lb., another weighed 200 lb. and the third weighed 300 lb., both groups have the same average (200 lb.), but the body weights vary much more in the second group, giving it a higher standard deviation: the standard deviation for the first group is 0 and for the second group, it's 100.

Given the data available in this report, examining the standard deviation of the angles is a quick way to evaluate how consistent the grippers in each group are, or to look at it the other way, how much the grippers vary. Remember, the larger the standard deviation, the more they vary; and the smaller the standard deviation, the more consistent they are, or the less they vary.

Using the entire sample, we calculated the standard deviation for the angles and it equaled 3.74 degrees. Taking on faith the grippers that had been identified as from IronMind, we calculated the standard deviation and got 3.07. What does this mean? It means that the IronMind grippers are noticeably less variable (and therefore more consistent) than the entire sample, which should have been the first point the author of this study noticed and reported. IronMind has been telling people for years how consistent its grippers are, and even if the author painted a very different picture, it's nice that this report provided data proving our point.

Next we took the grippers that the author had identified as from IronMind and subdivided them into two groups: those that were our Captains of Crush Grippers and those that were our earlier pre-Captains of Crush Grippers. Calculating the standard deviation for the Captains of Crush Grippers only, we got 1.58(!), which once again corroborated that IronMind's Captains of Crush Grippers had established new standards of accuracy in the gripper world.

Gripper variation/consistency

Group	Standard deviation of angle (degrees)*
Entire sample	3.74
All IronMind grippers (old and new)	3.07
Captains of Crush grippers only	1.58

* a larger standard deviation means they vary more, a smaller standard deviation means they are more consistent

The results speak for themselves

Thus, for all their obvious limitations, these data nicely illustrate the progress in IronMind's work even if only up to that point in time, and the evidence supporting Captains of Crush Grippers is crystal clear. The good news continues, because our latest grippers—reflecting our continued progress toward absolute perfection—are even closer to being absolutely spot-on.

Testing with integrity

Now that you've seen how you can learn something of value even from poorly-executed research, what happens if you start off on the right foot?

A responsible testing program can at least yield reliable relative indices so that you can consistently gauge any particular gripper, and it can also achieve requisite levels of validity, so that the numbers yielded by the test correspond to the reality of actually squeezing a gripper. "Huh?"

In 1993, IronMind reasoned that even if the idea of an indisputable magic number did not exist for grippers, we could develop an indexing system that would give our customers a frame of reference for understanding, minimally, the difficulty of one of our grippers compared to another one of our grippers. As things advanced, Captains of Crush Grippers have come to define the standard units of measurement for all really tough hand grippers and hand strength in general. Thus, the value—and the importance—of our relative indices have increased tremendously over the years, even if we continue to say, "Take all these numbers, including our own, with a grain of salt and concentrate on getting stronger by training with whatever gripper(s) you have."

It is possible to test grippers in a way that does give you beneficial insights into how hard they are to close. I was trained to be a research scientist, but lifting is our world here at IronMind, and we knew that to be useful, any efforts we made to rate our grippers should be in a context that was meaningful to lifters. Thus, anything measured in inch–pounds (torque) or pounds per square inch (pressure), for example, was useless in actuality, even if it might make sense on paper to a non-lifter. When was the last time someone asked you, "How many inch–pounds can you deadlift?" "What was your PSI on that box squat?" Have you ever seen lifting records defined in units of either torque or pressure? Of course not. Pounds or kilos are the language of strength.

Assigning poundage ratings

When IronMind began testing grippers in 1993, we knew that "pounds" was the currency we had to use to describe how difficult grippers were to close. Further, we knew that grippers flex and tend to move when under a load, so that any valid testing system had to incorporate this feature or it would yield meaningless data. Finally, we like to think that intelligent people are always driven by the KISS principle: Keep It Simple, Stupid. So what did we do?

We can simplify the description of our procedure so that you will immediately understand the basic method we developed in 1993 and have used ever since. Imagine clamping one gripper handle in a vise, with that handle parallel to the ground. Next, hang weights on the top handle until it touches the bottom handle. Do this carefully with IWF-certified barbell plates, for example, and you will end up with a reliable, valid indicator of how tough it is to close the gripper in units that are meaningful to lifters (e.g., 140 lb.). It gives you the flexibility to argue all day about where on the handle you think you should apply the load (always remember that you are dealing with a lever arm, so where you apply the load will influence the absolute numbers you get, which is one of the reasons we hesitate to attach too much importance to a specific number).

This is an oversimplified version of what drives the IronMind rating system, and it is the basis for how we developed the approximate poundage ratings we supply with Captains of Crush Grippers. While it certainly isn't the only method that works, it gives you an idea of some of the elements you should watch for in any system that rates gripper loads. Note that this is an empirically driven system, not one based on what a couple of people might think—but what happened when we took our ratings and compared them to what the hands-on experts told us?

Way back when I ran our original numbers by Richard Sorin, he said they were right on. John Brookfield worked in the other direction, and we had great convergence with him too, as John, who likes to estimate the pressure it takes to crush different things, came in at 160 lb. for our No. 1, 200 lb. for our No. 2, and 285 lb. for our No. 3.

Happily, we felt this closed the loop in verifying our poundage ratings.

Pounded by poundages
Given this, you might wonder why gripper ratings from one brand to another, or from one grip device to another, are so inconsistent. After all,

even though now you know how much barbell plates can vary, you wouldn't expect one that is marked 50 lb. to feel like another one that is marked 25 lb., would you? Yet, this sort of discrepancy is all too common in the gripper world.

First, if the grippers from Brand X are inconsistent, the numbers won't mean too much, and it gets more complicated. Even if they are compared to a brand that makes consistent grippers, the ratings will seem squirrelly because any patterns that should exist get clouded by the variability of the first brand—that's one reason why the comparisons are not so simple.

Second, frankly, some of the ratings you run into seem to have so little apparent meaning or relationship to reality that they might have been drawn from a random number table. IronMind regularly gets phone calls and e-mails about this because someone has bought an XYZ gripper that is rated at "300 lb.," for example, and the person can close it, but not a No. 2 Captains of Crush Gripper, which has a nominal rating of 195 lb. We explain how our rating system was carefully developed, is empirically based, and while not perfect, has proven its merit.

It also helps to think of gripper ratings as being like currency and while Captains of Crush numbers are in U.S. dollars, other numbers you run into might be in yuan or euros or pesos, or they might be just plain counterfeit, with no real meaning of any kind. For all of those reasons, you can see that even if something is marked as 200, merely knowing that number tells you virtually nothing.

The easiest thing to remember is that IronMind gripper ratings have meaning within the Captains of Crush family. Don't expect numbers from other sources to foot to ours in a meaningful way, and don't expect the consistency and meaning you find in IronMind numbers to apply to other grip products. In addition, we would urge everyone not to get too carried away with the numbers, any numbers, including ours, and to focus on training hard instead—your body doesn't know what the supposed poundage rating is, but if the gripper is hard for you to close, and if you persist, you will get stronger regardless.

You may also be interested to know that a test done years ago showed that the average man was able to squeeze 112 lb. of pressure on a hand dynamometer, a special device used often by physical therapists and orthopedic physicians to measure hand strength. The test consisted of one thousand males squeezing the device with their dominant hand . . . the average man with the 112-lb. squeeze would barely close the 100-lb. Trainer and fall short on the 140-lb. No. 1 Captains of Crush Gripper, which shows that the ratings of these grippers are well-devised and right on target.

From "Training with IronMind's Crushed to Dust!™ Grip Tools," by John Brookfield.

Captains of Crush Grippers: beyond poundage ratings
Returning to the question of how hard it is to close a particular gripper, Captains of Crush Grippers have become established as the gold standard of grip strength, and each of our different grippers represents a clearly understood level of grip strength. Thus, whether in Mozambique or in Michigan, everyone is using the same frame of reference when talking about succeeding with a No. 1 or a No. 2 Captains of Crush Gripper, for example, or their mighty efforts to conquer the No. 3 CoC or the No. 4 CoC. We noted earlier that going back at least a decade, we found that a really tough gripper was referred to as a No. 3, no matter who made it, marking the beginning of this trend.

In addition to creating the rating system for its CoC grippers, IronMind considered the major variables that determined the load required to deflect the spring, as well as those that further influenced both the actual and the perceived experience of closing the gripper. We came to see that as tempting and as appealing as it might be to focus simply on the raw poundage rating of a gripper, this could very easily lead to the sort of widespread confusion we have seen, and it also missed some very important information that determined the actual difficulty of closing any particular gripper.

We realized that IronMind's more meaningful efforts should concentrate on simultaneously understanding and controlling the entire cluster of factors that entered the mix, not only the spring, but also the specifics related to the handles, including the knurling, their weight and dimensions, materials used, and so forth.

Tied to our roots
With an eye toward that goal, IronMind continued to refine our design and manufacturing processes, increasing our ability to produce Captains of Crush Grippers that are more similar to each other than might have seemed possible 10 or 15 years ago. Not content with establishing this level of control, though, we next turned to our historical experience with these grippers, as well as to our extensive records, clinical trials and our data bank of comments from rank beginners up to the top performers in the field, and we set ourselves a serious target. We would define the unique territory (resistance level) of each Captains of Crush Gripper, and we accepted the mission of ensuring that what we produced in the coming years was true to those very special roots.

And lest you think this is mere sizzle, rest assured that there's plenty of steak underlying those words. In 2004, building on these principles, we began our most serious quest yet in that sphere . . . how to ensure that the benchmark No. 3 Captains of Crush Gripper you buy today, while embodying the many advances we have made over the years, is as true as possible to what the great grip masters of yesteryear faced in how tough it was to close. This might not sound like a big deal, and it's certainly nothing that's relevant to a product without the history of Captains of Crush Grippers, but it's like a having a replica of the Inch dumbbell, which is very true to the original, versus the Apollon Wheels used at the Arnold strongman contests, which are strikingly different from the original. If you want to compare yourself on the historical measures of greatness, you don't want a moving target or one with little relevance. You want something that is as identical as possible to the original on the critical dimensions.

The IronMind News column (www.ironmind.com) is widely read in the strength world and on January 20, 2004, this story appeared:

> **The 2004 No. 3 Captains of Crush® Gripper Is Available**
> **2004-01-20 06:37:47**
>
> *Just released, "the 2004 edition of the No. 3 Captains of Crush Gripper continues the IronMind tradition of continually working to improve the appearance, precision and durability of this world-renowned gripper. Even when our progress is subtle, we seize every opportunity to improve our grippers, so we have always said that our latest grippers are also our best grippers." An object of passion for many, Captains of Crush Grippers are the benchmark for grip enthusiasts around the world, and outstanding performances on them have been formally recognized since 1991, when IronMind began certifying people who closed the No. 3 Captains of Crush Gripper under official conditions. Richard Sorin was the first man certified as closing the No. 3, and he is also the first person who will receive the 2004 edition of this icon of the grip(per) world.*
>
> http://www.ironmind.com/ironmind/opencms/Articles/2004/Jan/The_2004_No_3_Captains_of_Crushx_Gripper_Is_Available.html

Exactly what happened is that IronMind put its shoulder to the task of dialing in the venerable No. 3 Captains of Crush Gripper. We understood what a universal standard of grip strength it was and we accepted the challenge of ensuring that what current grip guys buy accurately reflects the deep historical roots of this peerless gripper. So, we rolled up our sleeves, pushed a pencil over paper, tried this, tweaked that, measured, and retooled, and then we took the final step we envisioned from the get-go. Without saying a word about exactly what we had been up to, IronMind overnighted the first of these grippers to Richard Sorin and asked him what he thought. Frankly, you could have heard a pin drop as I awaited Richard's verdict: "It's not the hardest No. 3 I've ever tried, and it's not the easiest. I'd say it's right down the middle." Call in the fireworks because we wanted a strike and that was the exact call we got . . . we'd delivered the pitch right down the middle of the strike zone and we could not have been happier.

Calibration at last

By now, if all of this isn't too dry for your taste, you have realized the really big thing that had happened. In a great irony, IronMind—who had realized, developed and promulgated the idea of grippers as analogous to uncalibrated barbell plates, and who launched the lone voice protesting the confusion between mere measurement and true calibration—succeeded in developing and delivering a gripper that actually can be called calibrated.

This success has real meaning and value to you because these qualities we have described are just what you need to make the fastest progress in your training. If you don't care about results, it's okay to try nailing Jello to the wall; but if you have a real target in mind—closing the No. 2 CoC gripper, for example—dead on the mark is what you want instead.

What's between your ears affects what's in your hand

Thus far, every time we have mentioned differences between grippers or the loads required to shut them, we have treated the subject as if we were only discussing objective differences, i.e., physical differences, but this is only part of the story. The psychology of these grippers, which focuses on the subjective factors, is also very significant, even if rarely discussed.

For example, as mentioned earlier, when IronMind introduced the process of stamping the abbreviation or model name of each gripper on its handles, we stamped both handles. Later, we switched to stamping just one handle. Interestingly, when we switched back to stamping both handles, someone announced "double 3s" were something of an insidious plot we launched to deceive and swindle the grip world.

Anyway, the rumors flew, and we had people swear that the "new" grippers were harder than the "old" grippers; other people swore that the "new" grippers were easier than the "old" grippers; still others probably just swore (mostly at us).

Harder?! Easier?! The truth is that the only the difference was that now, once again, we were marking both handles. Still, we understand that if someone is convinced that one gripper is harder or easier than another, regardless of the objective reality, that is just how they will perceive it, and they will most likely perform on it in a manner commensurate with their expectations. Similarly, at least among the insecure, you can bet that anyone who fails to close a gripper will tell you that it's extra tough or that a gripper closed by someone else was easier.

To give you another quick example of how objectively irrelevant variables can influence perceptions of how hard a gripper is to close, consider the question that stumped you as a young child: which weighs more, a pound of rocks or a pound of feathers? Before you laugh at those silly little children who can't grasp that a pound is a pound is a pound, consider that while we have never done a legitimate scientific study on the subject, we found that when we initially switched from steel to aluminum handles on our grippers, some people who had both models swore that the grippers with aluminum handles were easier to close.

Putting a spotlight on this phenomenon, we found that, under carefully controlled conditions, if you handed someone two grippers that took an objectively identical amount of force to close, but one had steel handles and the other had aluminum handles, the person was likely to say that the gripper with steel handles was "much harder" to close. Why? Its dramatically heavier weight was probably associated with the idea of greater resistance, and that triggered the related expectation of greater difficulty. Intuitively this is a perfectly reasonable assumption, especially for a lifter, even though in actuality it is false when it comes to a gripper.

In a related way, some people can get overconfident about how accurately they can pinpoint the strength of a gripper, ignoring psychological factors that influence their perceptions and the limits of a human's ability to make precise assessments. Humans are not calibrated measuring devices (in the true sense of the word *calibration*). Thus, you would expect someone to be able to estimate how much another person weighed with a number like "about 160 lb.," but no reasonable person would expect someone to come up with a precise figure like "157.65 lb." That's the job of an accurate (i.e., calibrated) scale. Those who claim they can do this with grippers . . . 3.1, 3.11, 3.12 . . . are fooling themselves and a lot of others as well.

This reminds me of the time I was at a major strongman contest some years ago where someone asked what the deadlift apparatus weighed, and the response was, "We never weighed it, but we think it's about 600 lb." Next, one of the testers was asked to lift it, and he was quizzed, "Do you think it's about 600 lb.?" "Aye," he replied, and from that moment forward it was taken as weighing 600 lb., exactly. Uh huh, and I've got a dog that can climb trees.

Finally, just to show how powerful the psychological factors can be even with a very simple product, one day we talked to a guy who was convinced that IronMind loading pins had gotten heavier. To emphasize the point and to keep it fair, I personally weighed three loading pins for him: two old ones that I had been using for years, and a new one straight from our inventory. They all weighed the same, so I told him what the weight was and asked him to weigh the one he had that he thought was much heavier. He did, and showing what a conscientious guy he is, he reported back that it had all been in his head because the pin weighed what it was supposed to weigh, the same as it always had. By the way, lest you think this guy was some pencil-neck keyboard pounder who doesn't even lift weights, this was a well-known and very strong guy.

Things get noticeably more complicated with something like a gripper, and periodically we get a call or email that goes something like this:

"I just got my No. 1 Captains of Crush Gripper and it's so much easier than my friend's that I was wondering if it might be a Trainer that was marked wrong?"

After asking some questions, we learn something like this:

This fellow tried his friend's No. 1 about two weeks ago at about 2 a.m. on their way back from a bachelor party where he was not the designated driver and he thinks that he closed it . . . once. Today, with a clear head and a rested body, he attacked his new No. 1 right after work, really fired up to do well with it, and he did . . . two reps.

Not having the perspective of a lifter or a trained scientist, the fellow is unaware of the realities of variations in strength and the impact of different training conditions. He focuses on one rep versus two and assumes that this means one gripper is wildly easier than another. After we have established the basic facts, we urge the person to get both grippers together under identical circumstances and, lo and behold, most of the "vast" differences evaporate on the spot (see Chapter 2, "Misperceptions of variability" for more on this subject).

Still, anything is possible and as hard as we try, we're not perfect; but IronMind has a standing offer to anyone who thinks he or she has gotten a defective gripper to send it back to us because we will be happy to examine it and replace it if it truly is outside our specifications or substandard in any other way.

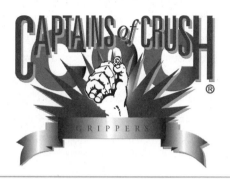

Chapter 4
Certification: World-Class Grip Strength

Captains of Crush Grippers: getting certified

Based on patent research that grip historian David Horne has shared with me, nutcracker-style hand grippers have been around since at least the early 1900s, and their appeal is easily understood. Anyone who glances at one knows what to do with it; they aren't intimidating in appearance; and they are portable, practical, and fun. Far from being a plaything, when they are as tough to close as a Captains of Crush Gripper, they can challenge the strongest people on the planet—which is why any place you see a group of World's Strongest Man competitors or any other group of really strong guys, you will find Captains of Crush devotees. What a great training tool and what a great way to determine who has world-class grip strength!

For many years and across even more miles, the whole idea of establishing bragging rights in the grip world has been closely tied to how people perform on Captains of Crush Grippers, and to lend some order to the process, IronMind started certifying accomplishments in 1991, when Richard Sorin was the first guy we recognized as having actually closed our

No. 3 gripper. Back then, the process was quite informal compared to what we do today: over the years we have had to add new rules and clarify the older ones, all in the interest of maintaining the spirit of the challenge. This is the same process that occurs in any organized activity as it catches on and gains popularity, and the expansion and refinement of our rules for certification stand as proof of how much things have grown since day one.

Incidentally, each of the rules we have is tied to a particular potential infraction and each can usually be associated with a specific incident, although we view each rule as a necessary precaution against violating the spirit of this challenge, not as an indictment of any individual.

Given that some of the pre-Captains of Crush Grippers that IronMind sold in the very early 1990s could vary in width and because some were just too wide for anyone with a hand smaller than a baseball glove, we encouraged people to position the gripper in the sweet part of their hand before laying into it with their best effort.

Deep sets
Over the years, life in the gripper world went on merrily and little second thought was given to this starting position. A decade later, though, a fellow who had come under the spell of the Captains of Crush Grippers wrote an e-book that was purportedly based on Joe Kinney's training principles. Since this fellow had only one brief telephone conversation with Joe Kinney and perhaps because he didn't fully grasp Joe's training ideas, the e-book had little to do with Joe Kinney or how he trained, but what it did contain—something that was central to its doctrine—was a starting position that became known as the deep set.

Thus, instead of starting off with the standard gap of approximately 2" in between the handles, something more like 3/4" was his recommendation. Following this advice, guys could more readily close the grippers because just as you can move more weight in a quarter squat than you can through a full-range squat, a partial movement on the grippers was easier than a full one. You can imagine how thrilled some people were to find out that they suddenly appeared to be 20% "stronger" than they had been only moments earlier when they had been using a legitimate start and were performing full-range movements.

Incidentally, if this development sounds reminiscent of the dark side of modern powerlifting, the analogy continued:

1. the new techniques were rationalized ("my hands are too small so I need a deep set")
2. the movements were mutated (starting positions became more extreme, moving closer to 1/2" and 1/4")
3. splinter groups were formed (everyone could be a champion somewhere on the Internet, at least)
4. suddenly the apparent accomplishments started to soar (the number of people who could "close" the No. 3 Captains of Crush Gripper skyrocketed)

The flash point for IronMind occurred at Odd Haugen's 2003 Beauty and the Beast strongman contest where I saw someone close a gripper in this style, with the added twist of keeping his palm turned away from inquisitive eyes until he had completed his effort.

"Huh?!" rapidly gave way to "not in our backyard," and so on February 11, 2003 we posted the following in the IronMind News column (www.ironmind.com):

> **Captains of Crush® Grippers: Certification**
> **2003-02-11 07:17:46**
>
> *Over the years, the rules for being certified for authentically closing an IronMind No. 3 or No. 4 Captains of Crush Gripper have grown in response to potential loopholes that are not in the spirit of legitimately closing one of these world-renowned grippers. Because of questions raised about the possibility of someone nudging a gripper shut while it is blocked from view and then turning the hand, showing that the gripper is shut, the fourth rule has been modified, with added language, as follows: "The free hand may be used to position the gripper in the gripping hand, but must*

then be removed, and must stay at least a foot from the gripping hand at all times during the squeeze. Similarly, nothing may be in contact with the gripping hand or the gripping arm from the elbow down (for example, the free hand is not allowed to steady the wrist of the gripping hand, hold the spring, etc.). At least the last inch of the squeeze must be clearly visible (the gripper cannot be closed while blocked from view and then turned and presented as already closed)." The revised rules go into effect March 1, 2003. The current set of rules is available online at: http://www.ironmind.com/rules.html.

http://www.ironmind.com/ironmind/opencms/Articles/2003/Feb/Captains_of_Crushx_Grippers_Certification.html

Little did we guess at the time that "the inch" mentioned here would come to take on huge significance in the grip world in another year, and while you might joke that an inch is a good as a mile as you just miss an unyielding oak tree when backing up your new car or truck, we found that one inch in the grip world could bring on thoughts of what it must have been like at the Alamo.

How this occurred was that between the combination of this language and the Pandora's Box of the deep set, what had begun as "at least the last inch" became, first, just barely 1" and then it seemed to rapidly shrink to something that was probably closer to 1/2" than a full inch. After personally watching a failed certification attempt at the 2004 Arnold that was launched with one of these sets, it was apparent that what had begun as a simple and well-understood test of strength had been distorted, tweaked and watered down to the point that nothing more than a lockout movement was being pawned off as a legitimate close. At IronMind, we had a very simple reaction: "This has got to change."

Credit card rule
We knew that the gap was just plain too narrow and that in addition, it was poorly officiated because gauging the gap was done by eyeballing the distance in between the handles, not using an objective standard, and we had seen some very interesting interpretations of an inch. The solution we devised came to be called the "credit card rule" because in identifying and establishing a universal standard, we chose that ultimate twenty-first century tool, the ATM/credit card.

Here's how we broke the news to the strength world on March 12, 2004, reporting in the IronMind News column (www.ironmind.com):

> ### Captains of Crush® Gripper Certification: The Challenge
> **2004-03-12 07:26:06**
>
> *Ever since IronMind® formally recognized Richard Sorin as officially closing its fearsome No. 3 gripper in 1991, certification on the Captains of Crush® Grippers has been a mark of accomplishment and well-earned pride among grip enthusiasts around the world. Over time, rules have been added and clarified in order to maintain both the letter and the spirit of this challenge. Responding to concerns about both the depth of the set allowed and the relative difficulty of ensuring that a uniform standard is really being met under the one-inch rule, effective tomorrow, the language of Rule 4 will be: 4) The free hand may be used to position the gripper in the gripping hand, but the starting position can be no narrower than the width of a credit/ATM card, and the gripster must show the official that he has an acceptable starting position by using his non-gripping hand to slide the end of a credit/ATM card in between the ends of the handles. Once this is done, the official will give the signal to remove the card and begin the attempt. Any contact between the non-gripping hand and the gripper as the card is being removed will invalidate the attempt, and the non-gripping hand must stay at least a foot from the gripping hand at all times during the squeeze. Similarly, nothing may be in contact with the gripping hand or the gripping arm from the elbow down (for example, the free hand is not allowed to steady the wrist of the gripping hand or hold the spring, etc.). The entire squeeze must be clearly visible to the official: the gripper cannot be closed while blocked from view and then turned and presented as already closed.*
>
> http://www.ironmind.com/ironmind/opencms/Articles/2004/Mar/Captains_of_Crushx_Gripper_Certification_The_Challenge.html

Some people were really happy about the credit-card rule and some were really angry about it. While it certainly would have been easier initially to turn our heads away from what was going on, we felt that if other people wanted to cheapen this feat of strength, they would do it anyway, and that made it even more important for IronMind to dig in and stand up for what we and a lot of other people felt was right.

The next day, we posted a follow-up item that had more detail on the mechanics of this rule:

> **Captains of Crush® Certification: Full Credit**
> **2004-03-13 15:52:56**
>
> *When we announced the revised language for the fourth rule for certification on the No. 3 and No. 4 Captains of Crush® Grippers, we might have failed to explain a couple of things clearly enough. For starters, some people have asked which dimension of the credit card is being used: the edge (thickness), the long side (length) or the narrow side (width). We are referring to the narrow side (a little over two inches/five centimeters). Similarly, there have been questions about the gripster losing momentum on his official squeeze because there is a concern that we are requiring a cumbersome measurement process that will be both time-consuming and distracting. Actually, you should be able to do this in a flash (sliding the card in and out), and if you want to hold the gripper in your hand unloaded, verify the distance with the card, and then fire away at it without any set, that is fine, too. You can also adjust your grip once you have been given the start signal, as long as there is no contact from the other hand, or the violation of any other rule, in the process.*
>
> http://www.ironmind.com/ironmind/opencms/Articles/2004/Mar/Captains_of_Crushx_Certification_Full_Credit.html

Still the same day, we addressed the question of hand size next, since IronMind got hit with plenty of questions and comments related to concerns that anyone shy of King Kong-sized hands was disadvantaged by this rule:

> **Captains of Crush® Certification: Hand-i-Craft**
> **2004-03-13 15:57:02**
>
> *Hand size has always been a concern to people when it comes to talking about closing our Captains of Crush® Grippers, and for good reason: doesn't it just make sense that you need a big hand to wrap around the gripper and that bigger is better? "Not to worry," we have been telling people for*

years, because certainly anyone with even average-sized hands should have no problem whatsoever getting his pinky on the handle with a legal starting position, and this is even true if the fixed handle of the gripper is moved away from the thumb base, toward the bottom of the fingers. If you have really small hands, you might have to be a bit more creative to get a solid starting position, such as taking the initial starting position with your pinky extended and only wrapping it on the handle as you pull into the range where it will comfortably fit on the handle. Once you have a legal starting position, you can adjust your fingers as you wish, as long as none of the other rules are violated in the process.

http://www.ironmind.com/ironmind/opencms/Articles/2004/Mar/Captains_of_Crushx_Certification_Hand-i-Craft.html

Finally, rounding out what had been an invigorating day at IronMind as we fielded a flurry of questions related to this rule, we made it clear that while we had seen a need to plug the dike, we were not about to treat anyone we had already certified before the rule change as a second-class citizen:

Captains of Crush® Certification: No Second-Class Citizens
2004-03-13 16:21:17

A dominant question following the revised language in certification rule number four has centered on either kicking guys off the lists, making them re-certify, or somehow tagging each name to give more detail on how the person was certified. The simple truth is that there are no second-class citizens on our certification lists. If we thought somebody didn't follow the rules, we would not have certified him in the first place, and anyone who has been doing grippers for a while or who has read the book Captains of Crush Grippers: What They Are and How To Close Them *knows that the certification rules have evolved over the years, just as they do in any sport. Our unswerving goal is to preserve the spirit, legacy and tradition that makes Captains of Crush Grippers and certification on them so unique. Not everyone knows that the deep set is only a recent phenomenon or that not everyone uses it even now. Some of the most recent and most prodigious performances on our grippers have not used a deep set, and we predict that a lot of people will be pleasantly surprised to see what they can do on a gripper without using a deep set once they give it a serious try. We instituted the one-inch rule a little over a year ago in an attempt to stop the trend toward deeper and deeper sets, but it has not worked the way we had hoped, so we felt that we had no choice but to act decisively to correct this situation. On the other hand, if someone wants to clamp down a gripper, leaving a gap the thickness of a razor blade, and then close it, more power to him. But that's not the way guys started closing our grippers for certification and it's not what we want our certification process to become. Having said that, we understand that rule changes affect the guys who are sweating bullets on these grippers, and there is no denying that these changes can be disruptive. We apologize for this, but we felt that the sooner we acted the better, and we are here to help anyone who wants some suggestions for how to excel within these guidelines.*

http://www.ironmind.com/ironmind/opencms/Articles/2004/Mar/Captains_of_Crushx_Certification_No_Second-Class_Citizens.html

At IronMind, we knew that this would make some waves in the grip world and that a couple of malcontents would use this as a way to pound us and that others would use this as an excuse to whine.

"Impossible," we heard, "my hands are too small." While we understood that lack of drive and limited vision, rather than small hands, were the real source of the uncertainty, we also knew that the guys who really could perform this tremendous feat of strength were very happy that IronMind was trying to weed out the pretenders. The same guys—the guys who were the real deal—also thanked us for not caving in when people tried to bully us into watering down the certification on Captains of Crush Grippers.

Interestingly, while the uproar was as large as we had guessed, we had underestimated the tremendous groundswell of support we got from the grip community and from the larger strength world as we got emails and calls from people thanking us for what we were doing, and as much as we appreciated that, what happened next was the real eye-opener.

Along with the guys who wrote to us saying things like, "Of course this is how you should close a gripper . . . That's what I have always done anyway . . . Deep squatters don't use deep sets," we heard the following:

"At first, I was very unhappy about this because I felt that I could not do this and I felt robbed. I knew that it was kind of cheesy to start off with the handles practically touching, but at least that way I felt I could close the No. 3 CoC someday. With the new rule, I thought it was hopeless, but then I did what you said and I gave this starting position a try and now I think I can do this."

Hallelujahs were optional at this point, but at IronMind, we felt that this was a real breakthrough beyond the concerted effort by a few guys to lower everyone's expectations and standards. The guys with guts voted with their guts and admitted that deep sets were for grippers you weren't really strong enough to close, and they eventually rose to the challenge of closing the gripper legitimately.

One last point about this is vital because it's another example of how what you think is true about grippers might not be true at all. If this deep set starting position matter is interesting to you and if you want an easy way to look smart the next time you post something on this subject, take a moment and read the chronology of events again. What some Internet gripsters describe as the "old IronMind certification rule," referring to the one-inch minimum, came into being 12 years after we launched our certification system and lasted only one year. The one-inch rule was the anomaly in the first 18 years of certification and proved to be an inadequate bulwark against a flood of deep-set attempts.

Without the advantage of this spotlighted summary, I explained the chronology of our certification rules to a guy down at Muscle Beach one day. He must have been listening intently or just was pretty smart, because when I'd finished, he said, "So the one-inch thing was the morph." I nodded, almost surprised that he'd grasped something so quickly that had eluded many others.

Further refinements

As part of the certification process, IronMind has gone a long way toward tightening up the refereeing and documentation we require, always trying to plug loopholes as they reveal themselves. In our very earliest days, for example, a photograph and a credible source vouching for the person got him on the list. When Warren Tetting told me that he believed Richard Sorin could really close our No. 3 CoC gripper and Richard sent us a photo, that evidence was good enough for us.

Now things are very different, as shown when we certified Nathan Holle on the No. 4 CoC gripper. Nathan was the second person to accomplish this prodigious feat of strength and we held him to the highest standard ever, all in the interest of shielding Nathan's incredible accomplishment from the Doubting Thomases. Nathan ended up performing the close three separate times, in front of three different judges (one of whom was an IWF category 1 referee), and to counter charges that the gripper itself had been tampered with, we also had Nathan follow up his effort by squeezing a factory-sealed No. 4 CoC gripper that we had brought along on one of his trials. We did the same thing with another factory-sealed gripper that we had provided to his official witness/judge on another one of his attempts. Even before Nathan had been certified on our No. 4, part of

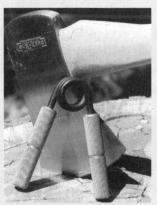

When someone claimed that the No. 4 Captains of Crush Gripper that Joe Kinney closed in his video was suspect in some way, we presented the counterargument in the 2003 IronMind catalog, with a photo of Joe's gripper and the following caption: "We heard a rumor that the No. 4 Captains of Crush Gripper that Joe Kinney closed in his video a) didn't exist, b) had been tampered with, c) was unusually weak, and d) all of the above. The truth is a) here it is, b) it's been well-used and is in fine health, c) when we recently retested it, it came in at full strength, and d) anyone who says anything to the contrary is mis-informed or has an axe to grind."

Reprinted with permission from the 2003 IronMind catalog, Volume 12.

Joe Kinney's documentation for No. 4 CoC certification included a video: anyone who would challenge Joe Kinney is encouraged to compare Joe's video to one documenting the best efforts of the earliest guys we certified on our No. 3 . . . since they don't exist, you can sense how outrageous it was for people to badmouth Joe.

By the way, during the months that Joe Kinney was training to close the No. 4, he was in constant contact with IronMind, telling us of his progress. Several months before Joe got to the point that he could regularly close the No. 4, he was hitting it from time to time, but he wasn't satisfied with his hit-or-miss performance. He wanted it to be a sure thing before we certified him and announced his staggering feat to the grip world. We were eager for Joe to succeed but waited patiently for him to reach the level of performance that would satisfy him. When Joe finally got to that point, we knew he could really do it—in full-range style, grinding the handles together lest there be any doubt.

Cutting corners
In 2006 we began to receive a number of reports about people who were shopping around on the Internet for the easiest No. 3 they could find—looking for a shortcut to certification—or worse, who were tampering with the spring to make their gripper easier to close. As a result, we began to supply the certification gripper, factory-sealed, directly to the official witness so that it could be opened on the spot at the time of the attempt. As with the requirement for the credit card gap as defining a legal starting position, this new rule created quite an uproar among the grip guys who were not up to this challenge but who felt that regardless of their strength levels, they were entitled to be certified on the No. 3 Captains of Crush Gripper.

The reason for this requirement was simple: IronMind started this certification as a measure of excellence, not mediocrity, and we figured there was no need for us to provide a watered-down certification, assuming that others would jump in to fill this niche—and that's exactly what happened.

On the other hand, beyond even the very nature of the Captains of Crush Gripper certification challenge, the care we have put into certification on the No. 3 and No. 4 Captains of Crush Grippers over the years—and starting in 2008 on the No. 3.5 as well—and the fact that we have plugged holes as they appeared in the dike has only increased the prestige of this accomplishment, making it the most universally recognized and widely admired accomplishment in the grip world. As in other walks of life, you don't get something for nothing: in exchange for its rich history and strict standards, certification on Captains of Crush Grippers confers enviable status on all who make the grade.

Gosh, and you thought you were just getting recognized for closing a really tough gripper!

Captains of Crush Certification: "Same As It Ever Was"

"I would like to ask what is the reason that the certifications with different rules are on the same list, without even mentioning that they are done with different rules?

"The credit card rule alone makes the performance totally different than it was before the credit card rule. And there have been other changes in the rules also, like new out-of-package gripper. It is like comparing javelin throw with old javelin model and new javelin model. Or comparing 100-m dash and 110-m hurdles. Bottom line: they are not comparable, yet they are on the same list."—question for IronMind from Timo Hänninen and Petri Hirvonen (Finland)

"A good question," we said, *"thoughtful, with good examples, and one that a lot of people might be interested in,"* so we decided to turn the answer into a short article because this is not something easily addressed in just a few words.

It began in 1991, recognizing a corner of the strength world that had been largely overlooked and a man who had done something most mere mortals couldn't fathom was possible.

Grip strength was the area, Richard Sorin was the man, and what he'd done was close IronMind's fearsome No. 3 gripper . . . a feat of strength that left many a big, strong guy goggle-eyed.

Back then, nobody really paid much attention to grip strength, but IronMind has always marched to its own drummer, and from the company's first days in 1988 it has focused on grip strength, recognizing outstanding performances in the area.

In those days, as explained in the book Captains of Crush Grippers: What They Are and How To Close Them, *the grip world was easily described in two words: Richard and John, as in Richard Sorin and John Brookfield. From there, what was a small, generally collegial group started to grow and things were uncomplicated, so when IronMind came up with the idea of certifying Richard Sorin's fabulous feat of grip strength, our procedures were quite basic: a photo and some back-up correspondence and corroboration, and that was about it.*

As time passed, it became apparent that IronMind's certification program for the most difficult Captains of Crush Grippers signified not just the most established and most prestigious accomplishment in the grip world, but it had also become well-known throughout the strength world, so more players joined the game. With growth, things changed and in their quest to get certified, candidates began introducing techniques that IronMind felt violated the letter or the spirit of the original challenge, so IronMind's job as good stewards was to plug the holes as they appeared.

Thus, rules were added over the years, but—and this is crucial—not to change the landscape, but to keep things level. We were, in fact, guardians of the status quo, the people who said, "That's fine if you want to start running an 85-m dash, but here at IronMind, we still do the full 100."

Briefly, the rules for certification follow the chronological order of their introduction and each is tied to a specific incident that created the need for that rule. As for the most recent additions, let's consider them for a moment.

For years, there was no need to formally define a legal starting position, even in the very early days when IronMind sold grippers that were a lot more variable than today's Captains of Crush Grippers—some had Grand Canyon spreads. This is important to understand because even though we used to encourage people to pull in the far handle a bit if necessary, nobody got carried away with this and thus there was no need to get too rigid about things, then. Enter Kinney Training Adapted *(shortened to* KTA*)*, Bill Piche's e-book on gripper training purportedly based on Joe Kinney's training, and things changed.

For the record, Joe Kinney said that Bill Piche had one brief phone conversation with him, and Joe Kinney can quickly disabuse you of the notion that this book reflects his thinking. What KTA did present, however, was a systematic gripper training program and its key was teaching what has become known as the deep set: encouraging people to position the gripper farther forward in their hand, turning what had been a full-range movement into a partial movement, and thereby giving people a false sense of their strength levels and a ready excuse to complain about the size of their hands.

Because of this, IronMind had to reign in the partial movements that were an insult to the people who could legitimately perform this prestigious feat of strength: we saw the deep set as making a mockery of things that had an honorable tradition. For one year, we tried a one-inch rule and found that didn't work, and then we adopted what a lot of people in the grip strength community call "the credit card rule."

As for the fresh-from-the-package requirement, this too was in response to changes in the landscape: from a known instance of a spring being switched to unabashed shopping around for "an easy No. 3 to cert on," those without scruples were trying to dilute the Captains of Crush certification challenge with their frauds, so IronMind responded by requiring that a factory-fresh gripper be opened on the spot, eliminating these loopholes.

So, has the game really changed? IronMind would say, "Absolutely not," and here's the living proof.

When the first man ever certified, Richard Sorin, who had done so under the earliest, most basic rules, recently re-certified under the most up-to-date and complete set of rules, it's hard to argue that things have changed: the strong are still the strong, and all IronMind has done has made it more difficult for the charlatans to dilute things. After all, we figured, they can still run the 85-m dash if they want to . . . just not in our backyard.

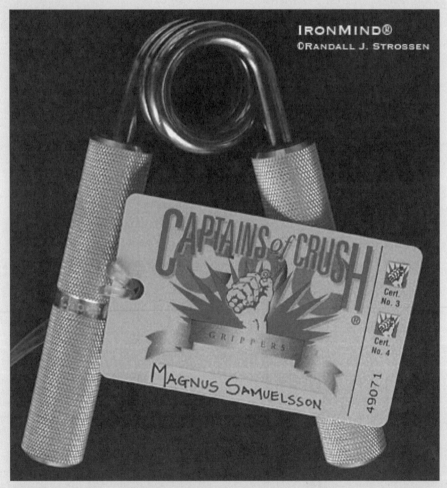

You can mash this and squash that, but getting certified on the hardest Captains of Crush Grippers is what tells the world that you are among the grip-strength elite, the men with the world's strongest hands.

Reprinted from the IronMind News, July 20, 2009:
http://www.ironmind.com/ironmind/opencms/Articles/2009/Jul/Captains_of_Crush_Certification_Same_As_It_Ever_Was.html

The legacy

While Captains of Crush Grippers adhere to very strict product quality standards, there is another factor that sets them apart—they have roots in strength history that no other grip device and few pieces of exercise equipment of any type can match, a sense of character and tradition that has been forged and honed over time. We at IronMind have always considered it our responsibility to be good stewards of this tradition, and we appreciate the many times Richard Sorin has commented on this.

Indicentally, this is why, for example, while always seeking improvements, we have never made any changes to our grippers that we felt would sever their link to this rich past. Therefore, when we embarked on our program for improving their precision over the years, we developed the guiding principle and goal of—in statistical terms—guarding the original central tendency while shrinking the variance. In other words, we design and manufacture Captains of Crush Grippers to consistently cluster in the bull's-eye of our target, which is defined by the standards established over these many years. Thus, despite all of our improvements, the unique history of Captains of Crush Grippers is preserved and reflected in each gripper we sell, even as we have continued our pursuit of the perfect product.

Captains of Crush Grippers: an icon in the Iron Game and beyond
When you hold a Captains of Crush Gripper in your hand—whether it's a Guide or a No. 4—you are undeniably connected to the world's greatest tradition of grip strength. Know that when you grab one of these grippers, you are part of this unique legacy, and that you are also connected with people whose world-class accomplishments go far beyond how hard they can squeeze something. You might not be an Olympic gold medalist, a Nobel laureate, a superstar professional athlete, a past president of the United States, a World's Strongest Man winner, or a world-renowned musician, but you would not be the first person with those credentials to train on IronMind's Captains of Crush Grippers. And you're also part of the club with members who can practically crack coconuts with their bare hands!

Part II

Captains of Crush® Grippers:
How to Close Them
by Randall J. Strossen, Ph.D., with J. B. Kinney and Nathan Holle

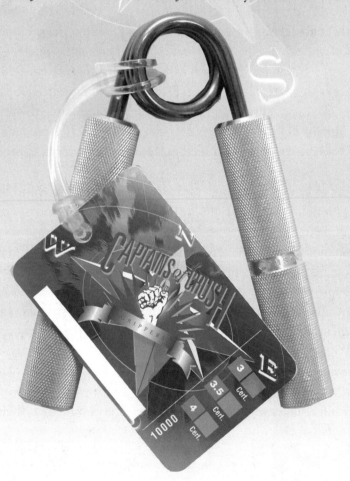

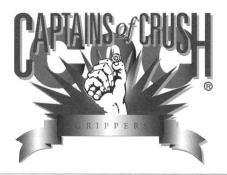

Chapter 5
Training Basics
by Randall J. Strossen, Ph.D.

Think: PR lift on a barbell

Most people were introduced to hand grippers via something from their local sporting goods or discount store: the familiar grippers with plastic handles and chrome-plated springs, cheaply made overseas and a lot of fun to squeeze . . . until they broke. Because these grippers didn't offer much resistance, everyone got used to the idea of squeezing them endlessly (and often mindlessly) as they drove to work or watched TV, for example. Unfortunately, it almost became a conditioned response wherein grippers were automatically associated with high-repetition, low-concentration training, and from 1990 on, one of IronMind's primary missions in the grip world has been to re-educate people in how to best train with hand grippers to increase their grip strength.

Moving toward this goal, the first thing we tell people is to forget that this is a little piece of exercise equipment that weighs less than a pound. Instead, view your target Captains of Crush Gripper as being like a barbell loaded to your personal record (PR) deadlift, squat, or power clean: treat it with the same respect and you will immediately be on the right track. To further help IronMind customers understand the basic principles of effective training on a hand gripper, we ask them to consider how they would train to boost their PR bench press, for example. If they were trying to bench press 500 lb., we ask, would they do endless sets of 100 push-ups day after day, or would they focus on a limited number of sets using heavy weights and low reps, adding weight to the bar whenever they could? Nobody has ever answered that they would do the push-ups.

Principles of training
From here we extend the lifting analogy, because now that you view your gripper as being akin to a barbell, you can apply the same generally accepted principles from lifting weights to what you do on the gripper. "How?" you ask.

Remember that the basic drivers for progress with your lifting are the **progressive resistance** and **overload** principles, which go back at least as far as the days of one Milo of Crotona. The fabled Olympic champion wrestler from ancient Greece gave the barbell thing a boost by carrying a calf on his shoulders every day as a basic element in his training program. The calf grew and got heavier, increasing Milo's load (progressive resistance), and because Milo's muscles had to do more today than they did yesterday (overload), they responded by getting stronger. This story is described in more detail in the book *SUPER SQUATS: How To Gain 30 Pounds of Muscle in 6 Weeks* because it is the basis of effective weight training; and Milo, being such a stellar strength athlete, went on to have the world's premier publication for serious strength athletes named in his honor: *MILO®: A Journal for Serious Strength Athletes* . . . a measure of redemption for a guy who ended up committing hubris and being eaten by wolves as a result!

Definitions
Progressive resistance Doing more in training today than you did yesterday. **Overload** Subjecting your body to a greater load than it's used to.

Progressive resistance and overload: if you remember nothing else when you train, you can't go far wrong. Add the principle of warming up and you're on your way.

IronMind's recommended approach to training on our Captains of Crush Grippers has mirrored this philosophy, so we have long advised people to begin with a program that is based on several sets of low-repetition training. Do a warm-up set or 2, followed by 2 or 3 work sets, and that's the essence of an effective basic training program. In fact, that is what we consider the core training program for everyone who is interested in boosting his or her crushing grip: do 1 or 2 warm-up sets followed by 2 or 3 work sets. Keep the reps low and the effort high on the work sets, and as long as you also allow yourself time to recover, you have no choice but to get stronger.

Core training program: 5 x 5

- 1–2 warm-up sets, followed by
- 2–3 work sets

Remember, it is no accident that the 5 x 5 program, with 2 progressively heavier warm-up sets followed by 3 work sets at maximum effort, is so effective for building strength on the big lifts. Also remember to think of your Captains of Crush Gripper as being like a barbell loaded up with a lot of big plates, and your efforts to close it should parallel what you would do to lift that bar. We'll go over the 5 x 5 program in more detail later in this chapter.

Taking this one step further, we suggest that, just as you would stretch your joints and muscles before hitting some heavy squats or snatches, you should stretch before intensive grip work, and don't forget to warm up. Warm-ups aren't something you can ignore: warmed-up muscles are less likely to get injured and more likely to produce maximum force, a pretty good combination of benefits.

While progressive resistance and overload sound remarkably simple and straightforward conceptually, adhering to these principles in practice can be pretty rough, and at some point you might stall out. If you get stuck at 10 reps on your No. 2 CoC gripper, for example, you'll want to try something completely different, like working with a plate-loaded grip machine, using IMTUGs, doing strap holds, or going up a level and doing partials or negatives. Continuing to click out reps on your favorite gripper won't help—you need a new exercise or two to get yourself unstuck.

Managing the in-between zone
Starting in 1990, IronMind began selling plate-loaded grip machines and led the charge in designing this type of machine for heavy-duty applications. The traditional machines of this type have handles that move parallel to each other, and in 1996, IronMind pioneered a new concept by introducing a plate-loaded grip machine, the Hardy Handshake, that was specifically designed to work like one of our grippers, but with all the advantages of a plate-loaded barbell in terms of progressive loads, static holds, negatives, and the like. A lot of people have benefited from training on this machine, but interesting to us at IronMind, most people prefer the guillotine-style instead.

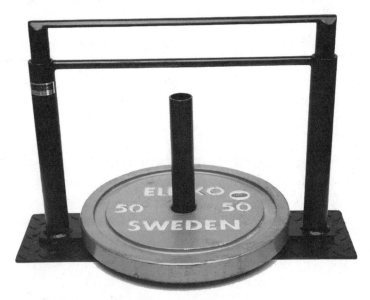

IronMind's Go-Really Grip™ Machine.

In 2002 IronMind introduced the latest generation of our parallel-handled plate-loaded grip machines, the Go-Really Grip™ Machine, the most advanced in our family of these classic grip machines to date. We had developed a feature that allows for increased range of motion in the closed position without pinching the hand, plus a new handle design that reduces the pressure on the soft tissue of your hand. Regardless of its exact configuration, we feel that training with a plate-loaded grip machine, not just a *mélange* of grippers, is the key to closing whichever gripper has caught your eye. Here's how that works.

Over the years, we have had people suggest, "How about making a gripper between a Trainer and No. 1." Fill in any two grippers you prefer and you get the picture—certainly a very reasonable request, but there are a couple of additional considerations that should be thrown into the equation.

Remember how IronMind introduced the gripper world to the analogy of uncalibrated barbell plates? Remember, too, how even with the impressive progress IronMind has made advancing the design and manufacture of our grippers, we still are quick to point out there will always be some variability among grippers, and the more subdivisions you have (along with the more variability you have), the more likely you are to end up with grippers that ostensibly represent different closing forces, but that actually overlap.

We recognize that some people just like to collect grippers—any and all grippers—which is fine, and that some people are perfectly happy to work with nothing more than the established models within the Captains of Crush Gripper line, which is also fine. Others would like to have alternative ways to progressively manipulate the load in their quest to move up the ladder of Captains of Crush Grippers. For these people, especially if they are very serious about their grip work, we think a plate-loaded grip machine is a far superior choice to accumulating a pile of supposedly intermediate grippers. The plate-loaded grip machine, besides being more effective in offering fine gradations of resistance, is more versatile and ends up being cheaper to boot. Anyway, that's enough talk, let's get back to squeezing the daylights out of your grippers.

Training principles

Beginning roughly two decades ago, one of the biggest challenges IronMind faced in educating people on effective gripper training was to disabuse them of the idea that the way they clicked out reps on wimpy grippers—mindlessly and with little gain—was not the way to go for big gains in strength.

IronMind is unique—and very fortunate—to be immersed in multiple specialites of the strength world at the highest level, giving us a perspective that could bring a lot of benefits to grip training. We have learned from other forms of strength training and applied this knowledge to grippers, always emphasizing the generally accepted principles of strength training to grippers. Thus, instead of advocating voodoo about dog legs and seasoning, for example, or shortcuts with partial movements or "easy" grippers, IronMind has focused on the things that have been proven to increase strength regardless of the medium. Our goal was simple: bring world-class strength training to the grip(per) world.

Thus, IronMind recommends such basic tenets as proper warm-ups, progressively heavier loads, a focus on full-range of movements, adequate recovery, a positive mental outlook, recording one's training, setting goals, achieving muscle balance, and buttressing the weak links in the chain of power. Let's look at each of these, and then develop some training programs that incorporate these principles: consider this a user's guide to new personal records in your gripper training.

Generally accepted principles of strength training

- set goals
- always stretch as needed, warm up, and cool down
- train progressively
- focus on full-range movements
- allow for adequate recovery in between workouts
- keep a positive mental outlook
- focus on intensity (quality), not volume (quantity)
- keep a training log
- develop muscle balance
- strengthen weak links
- take responsibility for your training

Setting goals

Goal-setting is essential to making progress, with proven psychological underpinnings and with real-world payouts. You need to know what you want to accomplish so that you can make a plan to get there. Set a clear-cut goal, with the benchmark defined in terms of both the accomplishment and the time when it will take place. A goal that fails both of these criteria is something like, "I want to improve my grip." A goal that meets both of these criteria is something like, "I want to be able to do 10 full reps with a No. 1 Captains of Crush Gripper by March 24."

If you want to get a notch more sophisticated about it, use a multi-staged approach that incorporates goals set over different periods of time. For example: "I want to hit 10 full reps on the No. 1 Captains of Crush Gripper this week; I want to close a No. 2 by June of this year; and I want to be certified on a No. 3 Captains of Crush Gripper by Christmas!"

Warm-ups

Force a cold muscle to perform and two things will happen: 1) you will perform at a sub-maximal level, and 2) you will boost your chances of injury. These things might seem obvious to anyone who, for example, can deadlift a quarter ton or more, but how often have you seen someone pick up a gripper that is at or beyond his limit and try it, stone cold?

Repeatedly, perhaps. Of course, some people can train like this, stay healthy and get stronger, but most people will not find this effective: the cold muscles will depress their performances for physiological reasons and the lack of progress will further slow things down for psychological reasons. If you get injured along the way, medical reasons will deepen the downswing in your performance level.

Instead, warm up before tackling a maximum gripper effort just as you would for a big deadlift. If you are just starting off, your warm-up won't require any fancy equipment. Sure you can buy an easier Captains of Crush Gripper if you would like, but you could also use a cheap import or a rubber ball, or you can even crumple a sheet of newspaper with one hand. As your strength increases, you will need to take the next step in your warm-ups and make them progressive. Just as a six-plate squatter might do warm-up sets with one, two, three, four, and five plates on the bar, someone who is training on the No. 3 or the No. 4 Captains of Crush Gripper might work his way up from the Trainer, through the No. 1, No. 2 and No. 2.5 before hitting the No. 3, and someone who is working on the No. 4 might well do sets with all these grippers, followed by the No. 3.5 and then the fearsome No. 4.

It's been said in lifting that if you don't have time to warm up, you don't have time to train, and the same thing is true for grippers.

Also, stretch as necessary—this can be done before, after and in between workouts—and include some form of cool-down as well.

Progressive loads
York Barbell founder Bob Hoffman used to say that if you lift 200 lb., you become strong enough to lift 200 lb. While part of his message was that you need to push to progress, another part of it is that you shouldn't expect to lift more than you do. Or as my junior high physical education teacher used to say, "You have to do more push-ups than you can if you want to get stronger." Joe Kinney's section on training is a graphic lesson in the need to push yourself, and my favorite is his observation, "That's why they call it 'making progress.'"

This is where the progressive resistance principle of training comes in. You need to add resistance incrementally if you want to get stronger, and while we at IronMind have never been zealous advocates of the micro-loading concept, we are huge fans of progressive resistance. Milo's calf got heavier, and by continuing to carry it, Milo got stronger. Your job is easier because you have a range of grippers to work with as well as a host of specialized training tools that help fill in the gaps, giving you the precise level of resistance required for your optimal progress.

Full range of movement
We know a couple of really strong guys who do partial movements and we know tons of really strong guys who do full-range movements. And while it's lovely to know that you can pull a ton or two in a partial deadlift, how does it make you feel to find that you can't move 700 lb. off the ground? Further, full-range movements lend themselves to a broader generalization gradient, which in ordinary English means that if you do full-range movements, the strength you develop will transfer to more applications.

Earlier, the deep set was mentioned: it's a partial movement with a gripper that involves only closing it the last 1/2" or 3/4" (less than a couple of centimeters for our metrically inclined friends). The deep set is the child of politics and egos and it is a stepchild in the world of strength. Besides being a parody of the actual movement (fully closing a gripper), it shortchanges the user in strength and then makes up for this deficiency by amplifying injuries. Here's how that bad combination works.

There are deep-set guys who say they can "close" a No. 3 Captains of Crush Gripper but who lift little more than Girl Scout weights on the Rolling Thunder®, a worldwide standard for testing a more open-hand form of grip strength. Once I sought input from Odd Haugen, a standout figure in strongman and one of the world's top performers in a number of feats of grip strength, even though he's as far from a grip specialist as you can imagine: "Why are these guys so bad on the Rolling Thunder?" I asked. Odd's a polite guy, or maybe he's just easier on people he outweighs by 100 lb., but I could tell he thought it was a stupid question. "Because they're not strong," he roared.

Guys who do little but deep set grippers get good at that and little else, and like the big partial deadlifter, they're likely to be red-faced and disappointed if they have to really close a tough gripper, let alone try their hand at a related feat of grip strength.

The injury thing is a big consideration because while IronMind has not signed on with the "dangerous exercise" brigade, we are quick to remind people that safety is always your number one priority because nothing will slow down your progress like an injury. We know of a gripper training program that specializes in partial movements and, jokes aside, it's no accident that this program has the world record for producing injuries: from soft tissue damage, to painful muscles, joints and connective tissue, to extreme cases where the person has difficulty fully opening his hand. It's not a pretty sight and besides that, it's not a good way to get stronger.

There's a reason why we have the range of motion that we do: use it when you train and you'll be glad that you did.

Adequate recovery
Training is traumatic. It's not just those nightmares you might have the night before a gruesome round of 20-rep squats or the anticipation of your certification attempt on the No. 3 Captains of Crush Gripper, it's also such things as the micro-tears in your muscles that heavy training produces. You are, after all, battering your body because, marvelous creation that it is, especially when properly cared for, it will rebuild itself stronger than it was before. And the "properly cared for" component is what recovery is all about.

In the mid-1960s, only the strength world cognoscenti had heard of anabolic steroids, but in the twenty-first century, the story of steroids is so well-known and so hackneyed that it's only a matter of time before someone markets his new electric toothbrush as "your old toothbrush on steroids." Steroids were called "restoratives" in classic Eastern Bloc training literature because a big part of how they produce gains is by artificially speeding recovery. We want you to be 100% clean, and the goal of adequate recovery remains essential when training your grip: it involves nutrition, garden-variety rest, and so-called active rest.

The human body is amazing: look at the junk some people cram into their bodies and yet they continue to function, at whatever level, for years. Try doing that with a machine and see where you get. Eat smart: protein, vitamins and minerals help your body rebuild, and rebuilding is the precursor to greater strength.

That's the fuel side, but there's also a need to allow the regenerative processes to do their work and that's where rest—traditional and active—comes in. Traditional rest involves some people's favorite activity—sleeping—which is the spawning ground of restoration. A couple of times I had the privilege of hearing a reputed insider tell us "Bulgarian training secrets," and one of the things he mentioned in passing was that sleep was unsurpassed as an aid to restoration. Wonder why guys who lift, lift, lift also sleep, sleep, sleep? It's because all that sleep allows them to recover faster so they can lift more—heavier and more often.

Active rest is an alien concept to most people, who simply head for the couch at the first sign of sore muscles, a big mistake. Instead, take advantage of your body's ability to buffer the toxic by-products of heavy training, which when facilitated by increased circulation is what active rest produces. Rather than becoming inert on your rest days, include some related movements—not heroic stuff, but things that move your body to speed up your recuperation. For example, the IronMind EGG was designed to improve on the proven tradition of squeezing a sponge rubber ball for your grip and forearm. Our feeling was that while the EGG could certainly be used for maximum efforts, it was also a superb tool for doing some lower-intensity training that would fit the bill perfectly for active rest . . . doing something very similar to the target movement, but at loads that hastened recovery rather than slowing it down. In addition, since we were designing this tool from the ground up, we tried different sizes and shapes, as well as different durometers (a measure of how hard rubber-like

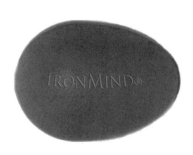

The IronMind EGG comes in two strengths: the moderately firm blue EGG and the softer green EGG that has more give.

materials are), until we came up with what we felt was the correct combination. As an active rest tool, the IronMind EGG is squeezed at moderate levels on the off days, with something like 2 to 4 sets of 15 reps being an example of an effective training routine for active rest.

Besides its physical benefits, active rest provides enormous psychological benefits, and the mind, we will see, plays no small part in your success with grippers.

Positive mental outlook
Thinking you can do something won't guarantee that you will, but it is a tremendous aid—and thinking that you will fail is an amazingly effective way to do precisely that. Your outlook is part of the psychological equation and it's the one you're used to hearing about, but there's more going on in between your ears that determines whether you have air between the handles of your gripper or are grinding them together, metal on metal.

Expectation, the outcome you think is likely, drives motivation: if you anticipate failure, your efforts will be half-hearted. Being rational, why would you put 100% effort into something you think will result in nothing anyway? If you sense the likelihood of success, though, you will give it your all, digging deep inside yourself for that little extra that will put you over the top. So, "I think I can" is a key factor in your success with grippers, just as in other forms of strength. All the whining about hand size used as a rationalization for why you must use a deep-set starting position is counterproductive psychologically: it's a negative perspective that will diminish your efforts. If you can pick up a Trainer and close it, but have to deep set a No. 3, the truth is evident: it's lack of strength, not hand size, that's the real factor. When you tell yourself lies about this, it creates inner turmoil that robs you of the psychological resources needed to mount your best effort. And, ironically, the more you cave in to this myth, the worse things get because you focus your energy—both psychological and physical—on the very things that are least productive for making progress.

Taking things in the opposite direction, IronMind advocates using psychological processes in a constructive way, employing the mind to help lead you and drive you to your goals. For example, one of the reasons we encourage people to end their training with a gripper they can fully close is because we want to reinforce the expectation of success. We want you to expect to close a gripper when you pick it up. It's the same thing when you focus on full-range reps: you get a psychological as well as a physical benefit.

Patience and persistence are the watchwords we often use to describe a successful training philosophy. Rome wasn't built in a day, and even though the Internet has delivered a nanosecond digital world to our fingertips, in the world of strength things take time to blossom. The ability to stick with tasks for a long time is a sign of psychological maturity, and it must be cultivated, so make this a part of your training philosophy. Similarly, persistence, the ability to stick with things especially through adversity, is also a quality that requires maturity and is essential to significant success. If you quit things after not reaching your goals in a short time, you're not likely to ever achieve much.

Focus on intensity, not volume
The traditional way of training on grippers—high reps—was necessary in the days when the only grippers you could buy were really easy to close and the only way you could get tired was to do hundreds of reps. That's what we mean by high-volume training, especially if there are frequent training sessions—sets of 100 reps throughout the day every day, for example.

On the other hand, training at a high percentage of your maximum effort is the key to building strength—that's high intensity—and it will automatically mean that you can't do too many reps. Also, this type of training tends to limit the frequency of your workouts, so that further contains the amount of volume in your training. And that's the winning formula for building strength: focus on high-intensity workouts, not high-volume workouts.

Recording your training
Remember that fish you caught? The size of a whale, right? Memories are imperfect and as fish stories illustrate, they tend to embellish the facts.

While this might be okay for casual conversation or puffing yourself up, this is not the way to actually achieve more. It's like driving from point A to point B: if you don't care whether you end up in Chicago or Baton Rouge, then road signs are of little importance, but if you really want to reach your goal, you need clear honest feedback telling you whether you are going the right direction and getting closer to your destination and so forth—and that's where a training log comes in.

Write down what you do each workout—not just the movement, the reps, and the sets, but also some comments on how you felt and what you learned. Then, go the next step and learn from what is taking place. Does one thing work better than another? Are there patterns in your training cycle that can help you in the future? Can you draw inspiration and added motivation by reviewing the ground you have already covered?

Some of you have probably read what I have written in the past about the potent psychological benefits of recording what you do in training. I have been lucky enough to see the actual training diaries of some of the most famous weightlifters in the history of the sport: detailed notebooks listing every weight, rep, and set done, in some cases leading up to an Olympic gold medal. Tommy Kono, the fabulous weightlifter, has notebooks containing the written records of every lift he made in his career, which included medals in

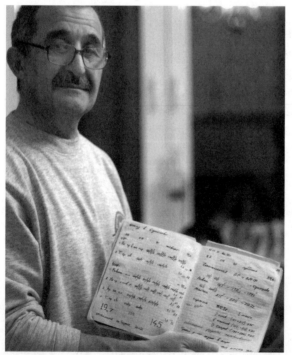

Weightlifting coach supreme Ivane Grikurovi holds the training log of his star pupil, three-time Olympic gold medalist Kakhi Kakhiashvili.

three Olympic Games. The fact that such great champions have such meticulous records is no accident: the training log is an invaluable tool for helping them reach their goals. And don't think that training logs are a passive record of the bare facts. I have seen training logs with such detail of what is taking place that a trained scientist would be impressed with the level of data analysis.

For some, training logs are intensely personal and they are no more likely to be shared publicly than a daily diary of your innermost thoughts. On the other hand, in the Internet age, it's easy to share your training logs with an on-line community of like-minded individuals who can see what you've been doing and cast their votes on your training, commenting on what is working well for you and what might be improved.

Muscle balance
There have long been one-muscle or one-lift specialists—the guy who comes to the gym and does nothing but bench presses or curls, for example.

In time, these people start to look decidedly disproportionate, like the upper-body kings with huge chests and giant arms resting on toothpick legs. Clearly, unbalanced development doesn't look right, but it goes deeper than that because muscular imbalance limits your performance and makes injury more likely.

My friend Tom Hirtz, who was a top weightlifter in his youth and who now puts his knowledge and energy into coaching the sport, once made me keenly aware of this when we were talking about lower back injuries—a common enough malady, right? Chances were excellent, Tom explained, that the back injury had nothing to do with weak back muscles; rather it was due to weak abdominals. The first time you hear something like this, it's a head-scratcher, but here's how that works.

Muscles work as agonists and antagonists, with the agonist contracting when it is the prime mover. That's what your biceps is doing as your arm, bending at the elbow, moves toward your shoulder. Your triceps is the antagonist in this case, extending as the biceps contracts. Having both sets of muscles strong helps you perform better and avoid injuries, as they interact in everything from stabilizing to providing decelerating force when needed.

This idea is only somewhat put to use by many lifters who focus on the prime mover on their lift of choice, and until recently, the concept was largely non-existent in the grip strength world—although martial artists have known about this for a long time. When you think of any of the principal forms of grip strength, and closing a Captains of Crush Gripper is a perfect example, your fingers are contracting, so 100% of most grip training is squeezing, squeezing and still more squeezing.

What happens is that by not training the extensors as well, you lose stability, are more likely to be injured, boost chances of overuse-related syndromes, and could even be losing the speed that could make all the difference whether your best effort on a No. 2 Captains of Crush Gripper ends in a click!—or a gap between the bottom edge of the two handles. For these reasons, in 2001 IronMind began to promote the idea of training the extensors, and we developed a product we named the Outer Limit Loops™ to provide a systematic way to train these muscles. We continued down this road, advocating muscle balance in the hands for both strength and health, and in 2005 we developed the Expand-Your-Hand Bands™ as another superb tool for training your hand's extensors.

Especially if they've been neglected, the effectiveness of training the extensors in your hands is amazing. We have seen that nagging elbow pains can disappear in just days. We have also seen batteries get recharged big-time as the complementary training revitalizes the person both physically and psychologically, and what follows are some pretty impressive personal record performances.

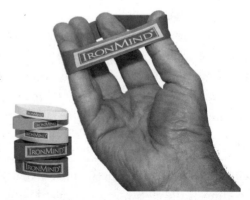

Expand-Your-Hand™ Bands, an effective way to train the extensors.

Strengthening the weak links

You might think that the line about a chain only being as strong as its weakest link is an idle cliché, but consider what goes into closing a Captains of Crush Gripper. What do you need in order to succeed?

Training knowledge – It can't help but boost your chances of arriving at your destination if you have a good map or set of instructions, right?

That's the role played by a solid training strategy and well-designed workouts. When people ask us for custom gripper training programs, especially if they are just starting off, the first thing we ask them is if they have read the training material that comes with their Captains of Crush Gripper—and most of them have not. This makes it easy for us to look smart because all we have to do is tell them to take a few minutes to study this material.

The next step is to consider such resources as John Brookfield's books, *Mastery of Hand Strength, Revised Edition* and *The Grip Master's Manual*, his Blueprint for Grip Strength DVD, and his "Grip Tips" at www.ironmind.com; Wade Gillingham's Grip Strength for Enhanced Sports Performance DVD; and most targeted of all, the training information in this book. There's also a lot of good information on the Captains of Crush Grippers website at www.captainsofcrushgrippers.com.

Dispensing training information can be easy for big talkers and the merely ignorant, so keep your wits about you, especially on the Internet. Does the person have legitimate credentials and experience to be giving advice that is worth paying attention to?

Motivation – All the knowledge (and talent) in the world won't do you a lick of good if you're not motivated to train according to the plan, so anything you do to fire yourself up can help to produce good results. Having the support of a group of kindred spirits, live or digital, can be vital . . . they can spur you on and if you're lucky, they can also be a source of sound advice.

Focus – Be serious when you train, which starts with keeping your mouth closed except when you want to take a deep breath for a maximum effort. If you yak when you squat, you should try shutting your mouth, slipping some more plates on the bar, and making some progress instead of just talking about it. The same thing applies on the grippers: close your mouth and close the grippers.

Details – Be thoughtful about the details. Most people get the big things right, but they blow it on the little things. If you are serious about making progress and have your eye on closing any of the toughest Captains of Crush Grippers (No. 3, No. 3.5, or No. 4), don't be cavalier about how you do any of the little things related to your grip training. From finding the sweet spot in your hand or having the right attitude, get the details right and the results you want will follow.

Take responsibility—no excuses
Don't make excuses or blame others for your lack of progress. In lifting, it's common for anyone who is beaten to say the other guy was taking (more, better) drugs, but even if he were, what does that have to do with how you are performing? If you're not getting better, take responsibility for your lack of progress.

Remember, too, that while it's nice and cozy to have a bunch of "attaboy" friends, this might not take you where you want to go. For example, it would probably be pretty easy to get on the Internet and find a group of people who believe the Earth is flat, quick to champion this idea and shred anyone who dares to disagree with them. But let's face it: all this proves is that ignorance or a massive blind spot defines this group.

Be alert to the same sort of process in the training and strength worlds. Sure, you can find a group that will support any fringe idea you fancy, but if your goal is to get stronger, focus on your own progress and take responsibility for your training when things don't go right. Beware of blaming others and be alert to how groupthink might be clouding your vision.

Core training

Earlier we established our core training program, which is based on the 5 x 5 model: 1 to 2 warm-ups followed by 2 to 3 work sets. This might then be followed by challenge work. The CoC training system divides your Captains of Crush Grippers into 3 categories:

1. **warm-up gripper:** it's easy to close, but this level is what primes you for the work ahead

2. **working gripper:** you can only close it for a few reps or so, but this is where you make progress, getting stronger in return for the effort you put into these reps

3. **challenge gripper:** even after your best effort on this gripper, there's still some daylight between the handles, and Joe Kinney would say that training on your challenge gripper is where you make your best gains, if you do things right

You'll know exactly how many reps you can do on your warm-up and working grippers—just count them. However on the challenge gripper, you'll want to be able to measure the gap between the handles and chart its diminishing size with accuracy. You need to be precise in the measurement so that you're not fooling yourself about whether it really was a quarter or eighth of an inch. For progress to take place, your gains must be real and exact, not "perhaps" or "might have." Use the CoC Key, which gives you 10 different measurements—2, 4, 6, 8, 10, 12, 14, and 16 mm along with 19 and 54 mm—to measure the gap precisely and record the results in your training log.

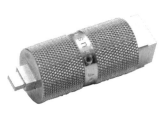

Measure your progress with the CoC Key.

A basic program might look something like 5 sets of work directly on your gripper, with the first 2 sets being progressively heavier warm-ups and then 3 work sets. Base the specifics of this framework on your own experience: for example, some people might prefer only 1 warm-up set, but they might increase the reps to something in the range of 10 to 12. People just beginning to train on Captains of Crush Grippers might begin with 1 work set for the first week or two, and then progress to 2 work sets for another couple of weeks at least, before progressing to 3 work sets if they even feel the need to add additional work.

5 x 5 program
Coming back to the 5 x 5 program we introduced at the beginning of the chapter, here's how it might look in practice. Suppose you have already established yourself as having an unusually high level of hand strength, as witnessed by the fact that you can click out a few reps on a No. 2 Captains of Crush Gripper. What would your training look like? You might do 5 reps with a Trainer as your first warm-up set, followed by 5 reps with a No. 1 as your second warm-up set. Next come your work sets, so named because this is where the effort you put out will drive the progress you make. This is when talking about progressive resistance and overload is replaced by doing what these principles require to earn stronger hands. Do about 3 work sets with your No. 2, and go to failure on each one.

We like to limit the reps on the work set to 10 or 12, and at that point, we would recommend that a challenge set be done on the next gripper up the ladder: you probably won't close it yet, but this is the time to start working on it. Later in this book, you will be introduced to advanced training techniques, such as the negatives pioneered by Joe Kinney or the partial movements favored by Nathan Holle, but for now we're going to tell you to just squeeze the daylights out of your gripper.

If you have a plate-loaded grip machine, use it to work around your grippers. For example, it is perfectly suited for your progressive warm-ups, and after your best efforts on your target gripper, you can do a couple of work sets on your grip machine using the exact load suited for your target rep range. Thus, someone working to close a No. 2 gripper might do the same two warm-up sets as the person in the workout above, followed by 1 or 2 work sets on a No. 2 gripper, but they could then switch to a plate-loaded grip machine for a couple of sets of full-range movements that bring failure at, say, about 5 reps.

With a plate-loaded grip machine, it is also very easy to do partial movements—focusing on the final inch, for example—as part of your training. Generally, if you are including partial movements, we would recommend that you finish your full-range movements first (on a gripper and/or on a plate-loaded grip machine) before turning your attention to some work on partial movements.

Putting together these pieces, someone who has first trained for a month or more on a basic program such as the 5 x 5 core program outlined above can add 2 or 3 sets of partial movements to his or her full-range training as a way to keep progressing.

Training routines
For a change of pace and to expand your grip workout repertoire, try the following training routines with your Captains of Crush Grippers and where noted, other grip training tools from IronMind:

Strong and Healthy Hands Routine

Here's the training you do if you'd like to get stronger and improve your hand health at the same time:

15 minutes, three times a week

Basic Captains of Crush Routine

1. Warm up: you can use an IronMind EGG, an ordinary rubber ball, or a hand gripper; do 10 to 12 easy reps
2. Repeat step 1 if you don't feel warmed up
3. Move up one level—if you warmed up with a No. 1 CoC gripper, for example, now you should be on a No. 2—and either do another 10 reps or as many as you can up to 10
4. If you can't do more than 10 reps, repeat step 3 one or two more times; if you can do more than 10 reps, move up another level and follow the same pattern: rep out if your max is 10 or fewer reps; stop at 10 if you can do more; and then move up another level, and so on

Strong and Healthy Hands Routine (cont.)

If moving up a full level in the Captains of Crush family is too big a step at any stage, use a Hand Gripper Helper or one of our bridge CoCs, a No. 1.5, No. 2.5, or No. 3.5, to zero in on the most beneficial rep range for building strength.

Here's how that might look:

Trainer x 10 reps		Sport x 10
Trainer x 10 reps		Trainer x 10
No. 1 x 10 reps	or	No. 1 x 10
No. 2 x 3 reps		No. 1.5 x 5
No. 2 x 3 reps		No. 1.5 x 5
No. 2 x 3 reps		No. 1.5 x 5

Do this routine three times per week.

In between workouts to speed recovery, do the following on two, three, or four days:

- IronMind EGG — 2 sets of 10 to 20 reps of light–moderate squeezes, rolling the IronMind EGG around in your hand for different positions

- Expand-Your-Hand Bands — 2 sets of 10 to 20 reps, light–moderate effort, using a steady tempo on each rep

Advanced Routine

If you are advanced, follow the Basic Captains of Crush Routine (above) with 1 to 3 sets of strap holds, grip machine training, or one- and two-finger training on an IMTUG

No. 1 x 10
No. 2 x 10
No. 2.5 x 6
No. 2.5 x 6
No. 2.5 x 6
IMTUG5 x 5 (ring and pinkie fingers); repeat
IMTUG6 x 5 (index and middle fingers); repeat

Do this routine three times per week.

In between workouts to speed recovery, do the following on two, three, or four days:

- IronMind EGG — 2 sets of 10 to 20 reps of light–moderate squeezes, rolling the IronMind EGG around in your hand for different positions

- Expand-Your-Hand Bands — 2 sets of 10 to 20 reps, light–moderate effort, using a steady tempo on each rep

Advanced Routine

If you are advanced, follow the Basic Captains of Crush Routine (above) with 1 to 3 sets of strap holds, grip machine training, or one- and two-finger training on an IMTUG

No. 1 x 10
No. 2 x 10
No. 2.5 x 6
No. 2.5 x 6
No. 2.5 x 6
IMTUG5 x 5 (ring and pinkie fingers); repeat
IMTUG6 x 5 (index and middle fingers); repeat

Do this routine three times per week.

Gripper Graduation: The Four-Week Wonder

Tired of having a weaker grip than you'd like? In four weeks, following this program, you'll hit PR levels of grip strength and wonder why it took you so long to train like this. Wherever you are right now—maybe working on the Trainer or maybe it's the No. 3—if you are chasing Captains of Crush Gripper mastery and are ready to graduate and move up to the next level, here's your program.

1. Raise your right hand and say, "I will follow this training program for the next four weeks. Period."

2. Do 10 to 12 warm-up reps on a Captains of Crush Gripper that is quite easy for you. Repeat with your other hand.

3. Do another warm-up set if you'd like to.

4. Move up to a Captains of Crush Gripper you can close between 2 and 9 times*, and hit your maximum number of reps, remembering something very simple, but very important: all the strength you'll ever build comes down to how hard you work on this set.

5. Repeat step 4 if you would like, up to a maximum of 3 work sets. Remember: 1 really good work set is vastly better than an infinite number of mediocre work sets, so spill your guts on 1 or 2 or 3 all-out sets, call it a day and get stronger.

6. If you are advanced or feel that you need extra work on any of your fingers, move to an IMTUG and do 2 or 3 sets for whichever finger(s) are limiting your grip strength—keep the reps moderate for this and use perfect form. If you are new to IMTUGs, the chart below will help you select the right ones.

7. That's the workout—and remember step 1.

On at least two off-days per week, do 3 sets of 10 to 15 reps with the Expand-Your-Hand Bands, and if you want to include some active rest for your crushing grip, do some moderate-intensity work on an IronMind EGG on these days as well.

If you've been waltzing around your training or following some snake-oil system and think it's time to get serious, sign up for Gripper Graduation and let the Four-Week Wonder take you there.

*If a full-step Captains of Crush Gripper (Guide, Sport, Trainer, No. 1, No. 2, No. 3, or No. 4) doesn't put you in the right rep range, use the mid-range grippers (Captains of Crush Grippers No. 1.5, No. 2.5, and No. 3.5) and/or the Hand Gripper Helper to get dialed in for maximum gains.

If you're doing your work sets on these Captains of Crush Grippers:

Zero in on your thumb and other fingers with these IMTUGs*:

	Thumb/pinch grip	Ring/pinkie	Index/middle
Guide or Sport	IMTUG1	IMTUG1	IMTUG2
Trainer or No. 1	IMTUG3	IMTUG3	IMTUG4
No. 1 or No. 2	IMTUG3	IMTUG4	IMTUG5
No. 2 or No. 3	IMTUG4	IMTUG5	IMTUG6
No. 3 or No. 4	IMTUG4	IMTUG6	IMTUG7

*Remember, you can train one or two fingers at a time, although we generally recommend training your ring and pinkie fingers together, not your pinkie alone. Use this chart as a general guide.

All-Season Grip Training Routine

Sure, it's nice to have a CoC Caddy to keep your grippers close at hand, out of harm's way and ready for action. As it turns out, a CoC Caddy is also a *numero uno* training tool, masquerading as something that keeps your treasured Captains of Crush Grippers in line.

If you haven't already done so, arrange your CoCs from easiest to hardest. If you don't have a CoC Caddy, just improvise, even if it means laying out your grippers in front of you, left to right.

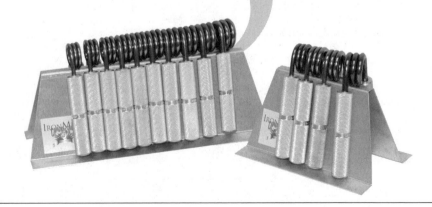

Warm-ups: Use with your easiest gripper, doing 10 to 12 really nice, full-range, flowing reps with definitive clicks tapping out each completed rep. For most people, 2 or 3 sets of warm-ups should do the trick, but you be the judge. If you're already pretty strong (legitimately closing at least a No. 1 Captains of Crush Gripper) and if you have a full range of grippers to work with, make your warm-up sets progressive: Guide x 10, Sport x 10, Trainer x 10.

Work sets: Next up is what we call your work sets. Ideally, these are low-rep sets with the toughest gripper you can close. Go for 1 to 3 sets to failure. Continuing with our example, your workout might look like this: CoC No. 1 x 8, CoC No. 1 x 7, CoC No. 1 x 6 . . . each set goes to failure, but with fatigue building up, your maximum performance keeps dropping.

Challenge gripper: If you've already been training steadily on grippers for at least a month and can do at least 10 reps or so on your work-set gripper, we'd like you to give your challenge gripper an all-out effort once every week or two. Your challenge gripper is one level above your work-set gripper: it's the next one up the line, the next one you are aiming to crush. On the day you do this, you will substitute this effort for your second work set.

This is how the whole routine looks:

Warm-up   Guide x 10; Sport x 10; Trainer x 10

Work sets   No. 1 x 8; No. 1 x 7; No. 1 x 6

Challenge gripper   give the No. 1.5 your best shot on this set; if you have a CoC Key, use it to help track your progress on your challenge gripper

If you are advanced, end this part of your training with 2 or 3 sets on the IMTUGs, working your index and middle fingers as a pair, and your ring and pinkie fingers as a pair:

index + middle fingers   IMTUG4 x 6 reps
IMTUG4 x 5 reps

ring + pinkie fingers   IMTUG3 x 6 reps
IMTUG3 x 5 reps

Especially if you want to try something different, you can also substitute IMTUGs for Captains of Crush Grippers for the main part of your workout, so as an alternative to the CoC workout above, you could do this:

Warm-up
index + middle fingers: IMTUG2 x 10 reps, IMTUG3 x 10 reps
ring + pinkie fingers: IMTUG1 x 10 reps, IMTUG2 x 10 reps

Work sets
index + middle fingers: IMTUG4 x 8, IMTUG4 x 7, IMTUG4 x 6
ring + pinkie fingers: IMTUG3 x 7, IMTUG3 x 6, IMTUG3 x 5

If you follow this workout and would like to also tap into the challenge gripper principle, test yourself before you begin this training cycle and test yourself again after 4 to 6 weeks on this program.

Thumbs up
Even if you're not aiming to chase Wade Gillingham's pinch grip performances, we strongly recommend that you do some targeted grip work for your thumb. Use either a Titan's Telegraph Key or an IMTUG and do 3 sets of 8 to 12 reps.

Expand-Your-Hand Bands
On your off days, put your Expand-Your-Hand Bands to good use:

Do several sets of 10 to 15 reps, with moderate resistance. Aim to do at least as many total reps as the total number of reps in your CoC/IMTUG training.

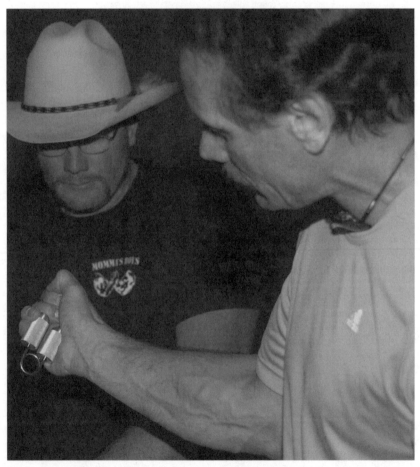

25-time world champion armwrestler Allen Fisher, owner of "the Fisher Forearm," was quick to realize the benefits of the IMTUG. How good are they? "Due to those things, my hand is so stinkin' strong that I can't believe it myself," Allen told us.

John Brookfield's contributions

An alternative way to layer another level of work on top of the core training is to use a technique called strap holds, which was devised by John Brookfield (see "Handgrippers: Closing the Gap" in the July 1996 issue of *MILO*, Vol. 4 – No. 2). This technique involves hanging a small plate on a strap that is held in place by squeezing a gripper on it: ease up on the gripper and the strap, along with the weight attached to it, will come crashing down. Strap holds can be an invaluable way to boost your final drive on whichever gripper you are working to close.

John Brookfield is known not just for being the second man in the world to officially crush our No. 3 Captains of Crush Gripper, but even more impressive, he's known for being all-around strong from the elbow to the fingertips, so he brings a unique perspective to grip training. One of the cardinal characteristics of John's approach to training is creativity, and that, as you would guess, means that John's training is varied, as reflected by what he recommends for aspiring Captains of Crush:

1. Warm-up – Go-Really-Grip™ or Hardy Handshake™ grip machine, medium weight, 6–8 reps
2. Rolling Thunder® – 3 sets, medium weight, 5 deadlifts
3. Captains of Crush® Grippers – 3–4 heavy sets, 3–5 reps
4. Titan's Telegraph Key™ – thumbs, 3 sets, medium weight, 15–20 reps
5. Eagle Loops™ or Claw Curl™ – 2 sets, light weight, 25–30 reps
6. Outer Limits Loops™ or Expand-Your-Hand Bands™ – extensor training, 12 reps per hand
7. Cool-down with Dexterity Balls™ – 5 minutes per hand

In addition, John says, "I did not put the Close the Gap Straps [for doing strap holds] into the routine. The straps should be used especially by the people who are gripper fans, trying to move up the ranks to close the next gripper but [who are] having difficulty. I suggest using these straps once a week during your routine after you are well warmed up; try to lift as much weight off the ground as you can, using the gripper and the strap, instead of holding for time, as this method seems to produce better results. Try the heavy lifting 3 to 4 times with each hand for the best results."

Later in this book, you will read about the training philosophies and actual recommended routines of the first two men in the world certified for closing a No. 4 Captains of Crush Gripper: Joe Kinney and Nathan Holle. Be forewarned, authentic Joe Kinney training isn't for people with a half-baked interest in grip training; and Nathan Holle's approach, while dramatically different, also depends on a level of mental toughness that goes far beyond the ordinary.

Finding the right training level
Our final two cents on your overall training is that it is fine to be concerned with overtraining, but our feeling is that there has been an overemphasis on the dangers of overtraining and too little concern about the dangers of undertraining.

When you train hard, your body needs time to recover: it is during this resting phase that your body will overcompensate for the rigors of training, and it will grow stronger as a way to meet the challenge you doled out. If you allow insufficient recovery time, it is correctly pointed out that you not only won't gain, you will regress and are probably courting an injury in the process. On the other hand, once you have recovered, if you don't reimpose a training load on your body, the insidious de-training phenomenon takes over. This is what causes you to slide backward when you quit training for an extended period of time. We find more people concerned with overtraining than with undertraining, and we think most people would make better progress if they boosted the quality, intensity, and volume of their training (our preference is for the first two factors, but the third will do in a pinch).

Having explained our opinion that most people are probably making suboptimal progress because they are undertrained rather than overtrained, we also feel that because Captains of Crush Grippers are so accessible and so addictive, overtraining is a real concern. Changing your clothes, getting to the gym, and doing a bunch of pre-lifting stretches and then maybe half a dozen progressive warm-up sets before you hit a really heavy weight in the clean and jerk is one thing, but grabbing your favorite gripper is quite another. While the effort required to go after the big clean and jerk acts as some protection against your inclination to overtrain the lift, the ease with which you can attack a hand gripper paves the way to overtraining.

If you ache, your enthusiasm is ebbing, and your best efforts are going backward instead of forward, you are probably overtrained, and the smart thing to do is just plain put your gripper away for a few days, or maybe even a week or two. More than one person has had a breakthrough PR after a short layoff: they were overtrained and when they finally recovered, their strength popped up a level as a result. Remember, don't mistake laziness or being a wimp for a legitimate concern about overtraining: you need to take your foot off the gas when it's time for a pit stop.

Which gripper should I start with?

Captains of Crush Grippers began with three models: the No. 1, No. 2 and No. 3, with each corresponding to a definite level of grip strength. People unfamiliar with our grippers sometimes have a hard time believing us when we say that most people who lift weights won't be able to close "even" our No. 1 gripper the first time they try it, but it is true. Our No. 2 represents a level that signifies unusual hand strength—we are now out of the realm of the ordinary and are talking about genuinely strong-handed individuals. Our No. 3 represents what we consider to be world-class crushing strength, and for two decades it has stood as the most recognized symbol of grip strength in the world. Our No. 4 takes things to an entirely new level, and in our thinking, represents the final word on really tough hand grippers—someone who has the hand strength to click a No. 1 for about 10 reps, for example, will barely move a No. 4. Sure, we could make even harder grippers, but until we see people clicking No. 4's, there's no need for anything tougher.

As often as a No. 1 Captains of Crush Gripper will stop the average person who lifts weights on his or her first try, we occasionally see someone trounce a No. 2 CoC on his first try. This is rare to be sure, but it does happen, and when it does, in our years of observation, it is more likely to be done by someone whose daily work involves his hands than it is to be done by someone who "merely" lifts weights. In 1993, for example, under extremely bad conditions at the Yukon Jack National Armwrestling Championships, the mighty Cleve Dean kindly obliged me and gave a No. 2 a try: he squeezed it as easily as if he were crumpling a piece of paper. Cleve wasn't a lifter, but he had years of farming and raising pigs under his belt, and his hand–wrist strength was about three notches north of formidable. Incidentally, John Brookfield and I have had a standing joke for years about the mythical flooring contractor, as our way of personifying the mysterious person someone else swears can crush—or did crush—our toughest grippers, but who can never be found when it's time to document the event. Please understand, though, that we mean no disrespect with this joke, because John and I both fully subscribe to this working hand strength concept. In fact, some pretty good advice for someone who wants to get strong hands is get a job where you're using your hands for something physically tougher than tapping away on a keyboard.

World's Strongest Man competitor Jesse Marunde, the first teenager to be certified on our No. 3 Captains of Crush Gripper, got his start in grip training as a kid working on his grandfather's salmon fishing boat in Alaska where he spent every summer. Part of Jesse's job, George Farren explained to me, was to sort the fish, which they would toss to him. At first, Jesse had to use two hands to snag each fish in midair, but after doing this long enough, Jesse developed the ability to catch each fish with one hand, something Jesse would later tell me nobody else on the fishing boat could match. And that, George will tell you, is where it all began.

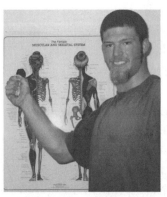

Tragically Jesse Marunde died in 2007, and to honor his memory and help out his two children, IronMind will donate $500 to the trust fund set up for their education for each teenager we certify on the No. 3, No. 3.5, or the No. 4 Captains of Crush Gripper. This offer stands for as long as IronMind certifies people on these grippers or until Jesse's two children turn 18 years old.

Teenagers everywhere: develop world-class strength, get CoC certified—and help Jesse's children in the bargain.

Photo reprinted with permission from *MILO: A Journal for Serious Strength Athletes*, September 1998, Vol. 6 – No. 2.

When it comes to selecting the right gripper, we recommend the following:

Choosing a Captains of Crush Gripper: 10 strengths for a perfect fit

Guide c. 60 lb. - the same difficulty as a sporting good store gripper, but with legendary Captains of Crush quality
Who is it for? Beginners, seniors, rehabilitation patients, strong guys who want an easy gripper for a first-set warm-up

Sport c. 80 lb. – now you're brushing up against the limit of what you'd find locally in terms of how hard it is to close
Who is it for? Guide CoC graduates, high school athletes, weekend warriors, strong guys who want the next step up for their light warm-ups

Trainer c. 100 lb. – if you're ready for serious grip training, here's where you go next
Who is it for? Sport CoC graduates, athletes who use their hands, people who have lifted regularly and want to begin focusing on grip training, public safety officers; an early CoC No. 4 certifier told Randall Strossen that this was his favorite gripper

No. 1 c. 140 lb. – this is where Captains of Crush Grippers get unusually hard to close—most people who lift weights cannot close this gripper the first time they try, and this is the benchmark gripper for having a good, strong grip
Who is it for? Trainer CoC graduates, those doing high reps on sporting goods store grippers; people whose hand strength is exceptionally strong from their daily work; if your safety depends on your hand strength, you'll want to get comfortable at this level before moving on

No. 1.5 c. 167.5 lb. – this is the bridge between a No. 1 and a No. 1.5 CoC; some people might prefer it and others might just grab a vine take the jump without it
Who is it for? People who would like an intermediate step between the No. 1 and No. 2 CoC

No. 2 c. 195 lb. – anyone who can legitimately close a No. 2 CoC has a grip to brag about
Who is it for? No. 1 CoC graduates and everyone who is involved in a sport where grip strength is a primary determinant of success should aim to conquer this gripper. Ditto if your life or someone else's depends on your grip strength

No. 2.5 c. 237.5 lb. – this is the bridge between the No. 2 and the No. 3 CoC, which can be quite a daunting divide between the merely impressive and the world-class
Who is it for? For No. 2 CoC graduates, this is the perfect stepping stone to the No. 3

No. 3 c. 280 lb. – officially closing a No. 3 Captains of Crush Gripper is the most widely-known and highly-respected feat of grip strength in the world
Who is it for? For No. 2 and No. 2.5 CoC graduates, and those who aspire to succeed at this celebrated feat of grip strength, certifying on the No. 3 Captains of Crush Gripper

No. 3.5 c. 322.5 lb. – suppose you've conquered the No. 3 CoC and are chasing the No. 4, here's what you master along the way
Who is it for? No. 3 CoC graduates, and those who wish to get certified for taking this big step on the way to the No. 4

No. 4 c. 365 lb. – certify on this gripper and you have proven yourself on the ultimate test of crushing grip strength . . . we used to tell people that unless they had a note from their mother, we would not sell them this gripper
Who is it for? The rare people who have strength beyond the level of a No. 3.5 CoC and for all mere mortals who want to get an idea of what the world's top gripsters are capable of doing. You might not be able to get a sense of what it takes to do a 900-lb. deadlift, but if you put this gripper in your hand, you can get an idea of the hand power someone like Magnus Samuelsson has

Overall strength, age, bodyweight, and hand size

While there are certain predictable patterns among different feats of strength, strength is very specific in ways that are not readily apparent to people who aren't immersed in this stuff. Thus, someone might note that there is little correlation between what one can wrist curl and how he or she performs on a gripper and conclude that hand strength is something of an enigma, or think that a cheating lift on a grip machine is a good predictor of what he can do with a gripper, which also isn't the case. There is no mystery here: different muscles or the same muscles used in different ways lend themselves to different results.

Thus, while it seems counterintuitive, closing these grippers can be pretty independent of your overall strength. Since our earliest days, IronMind has dealt with the strongest men on the planet, and we have customers with ferocious levels of overall strength who would be at around the mid-point on our grippers. On the other hand, we also have customers who have closed our No. 3 Captains of Crush Grippers who would love to be able to squat 300 x 20 and some who might not even be able to do an honest deep knee bend with 300 for a single (and yes, we mean 300 lb., not kg). Strength really is a lot more specific than most people would guess.

Similarly, the relationship of age, bodyweight, and hand size is often different from what might seem intuitively obvious. Generally, most people will do their best lifting in their twenties to maybe their early thirties, and everything else being equal, bigger and heavier people lift more than smaller, lighter people. "Fine," you say, "but now tell me something I don't already know." Fair enough.

How about the fact that grip strength is very atypical in these two aspects: age and bodyweight seem to have little bearing on one's performance compared to the major lifts. Thus, considering the list of people certified for closing the No. 3 Captains of Crush Gripper, as of this writing, we have teenagers as young as 14 making the grade, as well as someone as senior as Green Bay Packer great Gale Gillingham, who was 55 years old at the time he was certified. Richard Sorin re-certified in 2008 at age 57. As far as bodyweight goes, Jeff Maddy set the high water mark at 518 lb., and just as you would expect, we do have a bunch of big guys on the list, but would you have predicted that we would also have someone who was less than 150 lb.? Satohisa Nakada weighed only 137 lb. at the time he was certified.

"But how about hand size?" you ask. "I have small hands, so I can never succeed at closing your toughest grippers."

"Not so," we reply and we tell people that Richard Sorin once sent us a plaster cast of his hand(!), perhaps to emphasize what he has always said about how his hands are not unusually large, especially when you consider that he's 6' 5-1/2" tall. What might be telling, though, is the thickness of the hands. I remember how Joe Kinney, when he was on his quest to officially close our No. 4 Captains of Crush Gripper (which he succeeded in doing, and in the process, became the first ever to achieve this landmark measure of grip strength), told me how his hands had thickened so much from his training that he outgrew his work gloves and had to split the backs of them to put them on. And while people who are concentrating on closing really tough grippers tend to overlook their thumbs, Joe Kinney's massive thumbs have not gone unnoticed in the grip world—big, strong thumbs lend both stability and strength when you're clamping down on a gripper.

The care and feeding of your gripper

A loyal IronMind customer, the late Frank Gancarz, affectionately referred to his grippers as Papa Bear (No. 3), Mama Bear (No. 2), and Baby Bear (No. 1). When we first met Bob Bollenbach and heard about his gripper collection, we remarked that each was almost like a member of his family: readily identified, unique qualities duly noted, and thoroughly appreciated for what it was. Some really strong guys, we have said, sleep with Captains of Crush Grippers under their pillows.

When you have something this special, something you love this much, you'll be happy to know that this isn't a high-maintenance source of joy: save that for your horse or the exotic car you have tucked away. No stall to muck nor fancy carburetors to tune—just give the spring an occasional quick wipe with a Sentry Tuf-Cloth™ or a rag covered with WD-40®, 3-IN-ONE®, or any other light oil. This will block moisture and keep the spring from rusting, and it will also tend to keep your gripper running in silent mode, rather than creaking like your (grandfather's) knees or chirping like a bird announcing a new day.

The knurling on the handle of your gripper can clog up with chalk and whatever else it picks up from your hand, so take a stiff nylon brush and clean out the knurling periodically. We once got an e-mail from a customer who wondered why we had a problem unique to our No. 2 Captains of Crush Grippers: he swore that the knurling got noticeably smoother in just a couple of workouts, and he was convinced that the material we used for the handles on our No. 2 grippers was different from what we used on our other grippers, causing this problem. We explained how the knurling was probably just clogging up with chalk and told him how to clean it out, and that was that.

Gripper stamina
We used to get letters that began something like, "Wow, I am so strong that I broke one of your grippers." Gently we would explain that this was just a reflection of metal fatigue and that anyone could break a gripper—in fact, even in the early 1990s, when the life span of the grippers we sold was a fraction of those we sell today, we had noticed that our strongest customers never broke grippers. At some point, depending on a pile of specifics, the spring will just break, so always be prepared for that and always treat your gripper as if it will break on the rep you are doing right now. If you've never seen the broken end of gripper, let us tell you that it is sharp and mean. You don't ever want to have one of these make contact with you or anyone else.

Short of breakage, we have had people ask us if the strength of our grippers changes over time with use, and we have to say that under normal operating conditions we have never observed any change, and the most knowledgeable people we have met in the field have shared this feeling. However, if a gripper is taken past the tensile limit of the spring, the spring will deform, and this will result in the gripper being easier to close after the deformation. This bending is what is actually taking place when some people talk about "seasoning" a gripper. As explained later in Appendix 1, this is analogous to lifting bars:

1. You don't "season" a bar before lifting with it
2. Bars bend when their limits are exceeded
3. Bending could occur on the first rep or it could never happen—it all depends on whether the bar is loaded within its limits

We have never seen this happen to a Captains of Crush Gripper in normal use, although this is standard fare for the cheap imports, where 3" spreads turn into 2-1/2" spreads, and so on. Short of this, clicking out reps or even holding a gripper shut for hours (something we would not recommend) should have no impact on either its shape or the force required to close it. Having said that, even though we have heard amazing stories about the sort of punishment our Captains of Crush Grippers have withstood, we think it is possible to inflict damage on one of our grippers that could deform the spring.

Finally, while we have to say that we did not design our Captains of Crush Grippers to go beyond their normal range of motion, anecdotal data gathered from people who have filed the ends of the handles to increase the range of motion have not shown deformation; however, please be prepared for this possibility.

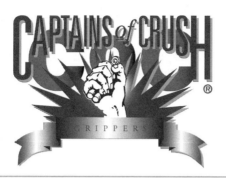

Chapter 6
Mortal Combat with the Captains of Crush® Grippers: How I Closed the No. 4

by J. B. Kinney

Having a 400-lb. bench and a weak grip is like having a powerful truck that can't get traction. So man invented four-wheel drive—and *grippers*.

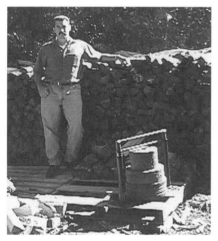

J. B. Kinney . . . the real deal.

There are a lot of good reasons why a man would want a strong grip. Tradition is a good one: whether you like it or not, men are expected to have strong hands. Worse than that, you're constantly being compared to older generations. This situation in particular is a good enough reason to be interested or concerned, or both. You see, there are some old guys out there who got stronger by accident than a lot of us will ever get on purpose. You'll be compared to these fellers—somebody's uncle, somebody's pa, somebody's gramps!—and there's no way around it; it could be embarrassing. I've seen some of these old fellers in action, and sometimes it's a very humbling thing to witness. It's not much fun to watch some old guy who uses a cane twisting horseshoes and squeezing them shut; even if he needs to use two hands on the squeezing, it's still tough to match. And then you've got to listen to how he's so weak now, and back when he was your age, he could have really showed you something. These guys are out there, and you'll run into one sooner or later. So, let's be prepared.

I'm guilty of it myself. It's great fun to destroy horseshoes and slam grippers in front of the young fellers. "Come on, son, give this gripper a try." "Hand me that horseshoe." "Here, let me open that beer for you." I'm just having a little fun, but it's easy to see the disappointment on their faces when this little guy with grey hair makes them look weak. I'm very encouraging, though, and always part ways with a kind word.

Another good reason to have a strong grip is respect: the firm handshake. You should have that. To some men this is very important and expected. Sometimes the handshake is a little contest, and you want to win every time. It's that simple.

I know a man who is a school teacher; he teaches auto repair to high school students. I have visited his class a few times. Yes, there are some unruly students there. Some children these days have very little respect for anyone. This teacher has even been physically challenged by some of his students. He challenged them right back—with his grippers. You know how that went: order was restored, respect was restored, and the pecking order was re-established.

Also, almost anyone, regardless of his age, can enjoy the challenge the grippers offer and even some level of competition. You don't have to close the No. 4 to have fun. Back when I first got my No. 2, I took it to work with me a lot. I didn't think it was much fun, but everybody there had a great time with it. They never got tired of it. Some of these fellers were in their seventies, some were teenagers. They all had great fun in their casual competitions. None of them was a weightlifter, but this was something they all could do, and they had fun.

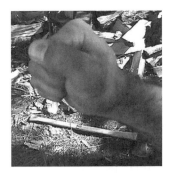

J. B. Kinney's hands are massively thick and strong—did chopping all that wood have anything to do with it?

Just about anyone can get satisfaction from working at grip strength. Age is not a problem. You don't need to be the cardiovascular equivalent of a deer. You don't need legs like Paul Anderson. Heck, you could be in a wheelchair and still have a great time and develop a ferocious grip.

Location is a good reason to mess with the grippers. You see, not everyone lives where there are gyms. Some folks live way off in little towns of 300 folks or so. Then there are the folks who live 20 minutes away from those little towns. With these fellers, sport is levering heavy sledgehammers and seeing who can hold things, like old car batteries, out in front of them the longest. These guys like gripping too. Most of them have destroyed every bathroom scale they've ever seen by squeezing them like grippers. The Captains of Crush Grippers are much more portable than the bathroom scale. Guys can stick a gripper in their pocket and they're ready to go. The urge or instinct to compete can be satisfied any time, any place.

A friend of mine, Tony Breeden, closed the No. 2 CoC gripper the first time he ever touched it, either hand, no problem. He never lifted weights, but he and his brother destroyed a lot of bathroom scales by using them for grippers. Yep, even with no gym, no weights, no machines, these fellers found a way to work out and compete. Funny how the competition turned to grip strength—maybe it's just natural. Don't fight it.

Getting started

If you're reading books like this, you've probably already gotten started, but give this a good looking-over anyway. Some of it might help you here and there along your road to strength. Even if you're an old hand at this strength stuff, you might find a useful tidbit in here somewhere.

If you plan to change your workouts any because of what you read here, that's good! You can call that restarting. The most important thing to do when restarting is to get a new notebook and make an honest assessment of where you're at now. I don't mean an honest assessment like we're used to doing. I mean a real one, one where you are judged harshly on your attendance, effort, dedication, and intensity. Do it as if you're judging your worst enemy's performance. You, of course, can't tell a lie, but he sure won't get any extra from you, right?

Write down your findings in the notebook and you're on your way. You'll be reading a lot of stuff about keeping score. Well, this here honest assessment is the first page of your new scorekeeping notebook. You probably already know if you're somebody who can make gains with low-rep workouts or not. Maybe you're the high-rep type of feller. Either way, high reps or low reps, you'll need to be using some serious weight, or in the gripper-only workouts some serious resistance, maybe not right away though, especially if you're new to grip work.

If you are new to grip training, you should spend some time on the light grippers. Stick with medium- to low-rep sessions at first in order to toughen up your hands. Doing holds for time is a good way to get the hands conditioned for what's to come. Conditioning the hands is very important.

The proper conditioning now may prevent injuries later. Your road to the level of strength that you want may be long, so be prepared. Do it right and get those hands toughened up. Some grip guys that I know have recurring injuries of the tendons on the inside of the fingers, right where the gripper handle touches the fingers. Don't let this happen to you.

You can prevent these injuries by conditioning the hands.

Remember to keep score even if you're just starting out. These scores will always be there to help you judge your progress.

Gearing up
First, we will be looking at equipment options and, later, supplements for training your grip. The equipment will not be glamorous and the supplements won't have pictures of skinned people on the cans. You're going to like this—let's get started.

You don't need much gear for this job. My own training was done on grippers and a grip machine. If you can afford a grip machine, get one, it'll help; its benefits are obvious, and we don't need to list them here. If you can't afford a grip machine, don't panic; you can make one or have someone make one for you, or you can just forget about it.

You're also going to be modifying your hand gripper. First, you'll want to file metal off the inside of the handle or handles of your hand gripper so that the gripper closes more tightly. Be sure you don't go past halfway on the ends, and watch what you're doing length-wise too—only take off what you need to. If you go to the halfway point, looking at the ends of the handles, you'll have a gripper that will let you train far enough past the range to make a big difference. This added range will be great for you. Did you ever notice that the gripper gets much tougher as you close it? Sure you did. Well, now, along with the added range, you'll get more resistance, too. Of course, now that you've got it all chopped up, your gripper's not official anymore, but it's great for getting strong with. Maybe you should get two of each, starting with where you're at now, on up.

I figured out the second thing you need to do with your hand gripper when I was doing forced reps or forced closures, I guess we'll call them— you know, the old press your hand down against your thigh and cheat it shut. Well, this is productive, but clumsy: you've got to be sitting down or bent over, and either way, after a while your leg is more beat up than your hand. The knuckles aren't looking all that good either where you tried to drive them through that denim a million times. After a while, you just can't handle it. Now here comes a very helpful tip: handle it! I don't mean just grunt and bleed all over yourself, I mean make yourself a handle for your grippers, a handle that will let you cheat them shut for as many reps as you think it will take. No more raw knuckles and bruised thighs for you, just very productive workouts with grippers. Now where did I put my hacksaw?

For the handle, you need a piece of steel tubing that's 9" or 10" long. I used a piece of one of those thirty-dollar barbell sets with the hollow bar. The tubing from this set was 1" outside diameter. The hole was way too big on the inside for the gripper handle, but the plastic sleeve that was on the outside of the bar looked useful. I cut off about 9" of the steel tubing and de-burred the ends. Then I cut off 5" of the plastic tubing and split it the long way. Now, this is where we get into some trial and error, maybe. On the stuff I used, I had to remove just over an inch of plastic the long way, on the same length as where I split it. The plan is to get the plastic to act as a lining inside the steel tubing. Once the plastic liner is in place, the handle of the gripper slides in and out and the plastic liner stays in the steel tubing. Perfect—not much to look at, but exactly what we need.

Now you need a place to use this handle. We don't want it to just be another thing we try to drive through our leg, right? This won't be a permanent mount; for me, this "place" is just a one-inch hole drilled into some heavy framework around a doorway in my little building. You need to find a place where the wood is at least 4" thick. When you do, you'll want to stand there and figure the right height for the 1" hole (yeah, make it 1", you'll need a good snug fit). The height I use is halfway between the wrist and the knuckles when you're standing there with your arms by your sides, regular-like. Drill there and you have a real comfortable station for forced reps. Using a doorway is good because you can get around it good—you can keep the gripper in front of you better than if you drilled a hole into a wall. A post in an open area, like a barn, would be great. Just having the hole drilled into a flat wall is the worst choice. When you start to bend forward to cheat the gripper shut, something bumps the wall; besides, you don't want your footing limited. Make sure you don't drill into any electric wires—that could ruin your workout.

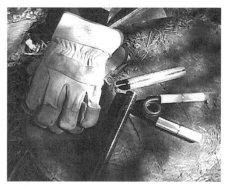

J. B. Kinney's weapons of choice (clockwise from right): Captains of Crush gripper, extended handle, leather gloves, and sleeve for extended handle.

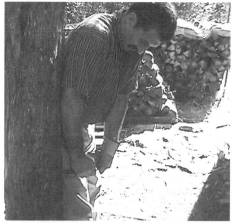

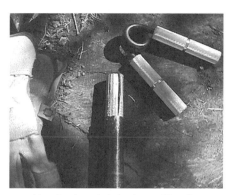

Here the sleeve is being inserted into the extended handle . . .

With the extended handle firmly lodged in a tree, Joe Kinney shows the proper position for doing reps, steadying the gripper with his gloved left hand.

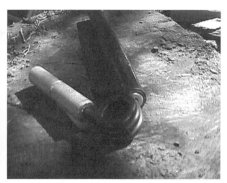

and, finally, the gripper handle is inserted into the extended handle and sleeve unit, for a snug fit.

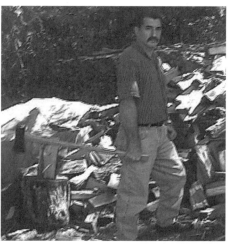

Joe Kinney can handle an axe—
backward and forward.

More gear: little things you can buy that'll help a lot
1. Black electrical tape: just tape one handle, the one your fingers will be going on. This will let you get more reps without the knurling eating all of your skin off—simple and cheap.

2. Wrist wraps help some folks, sometimes me—I like them. I wear them tight and loosen them during every break.

3. Liniments aren't just for after something is sore; they're great when applied before the work, to prevent injury by really perking up the circulation. Baseball pitchers get liniment applied before the game; race horses get liniment and wraps the morning of a race. In both cases, what they're looking for are the dual benefits of preventing injuries and improving performance.

Work environment
Let's take a quick look at your work environment. The work environment is more a look at what not to have than a list of things to get. First of all, notice it's called a work environment, not a gym. Building it into a work zone isn't hard: just disable the radio and you're halfway there. The idea is that it needs to be a place where you won't be interrupted by phone calls or people. That might not sound very family-oriented, but that's what is needed for the best results, and more importantly, for the prevention of injuries. The ideal would be a place where you could do your math homework if you had to.

Mine is a separate building, but a basement or garage would work, too. What "makes" it into the work area is me insisting that everyone leaves me alone while I'm gripping. That's all. After a few weeks, everyone will figure out your schedule and you'll be doing great. Bring your snacks and drinks, just like you're leaving to go to work. This isolation is a great incentive to get the job done. Sometimes it's a little hotter out there than in the house. In the winter, it's a whole lot colder. That's great, that keeps me on the job better and makes me want to get it done.

I've only been to a couple of gyms, but they were both the same in one way. They were both way too much fun: people standing around talking and griping about how there should be more benches to sit on. What a bunch of c***! Sure, there were a few men who were trying to get stronger: yeah, that's right, the squatters. The rest of those folks all seemed to be wasting time, playing with weights that were far too light. Maybe they didn't want to get out of breath as that would make it too hard to talk about football and hunting.

If they would learn to manage their time, they could have the best of both worlds. Set aside the time for your workout—do it—and then get back to your other activities. The boys at the gym talked to each other so much they lost count of their little workouts: "Did I do two sets or three?" they were asking each other. If they put some weight on the bar, they might notice. The correct work environment will leave you with very little to do other than to work out.

Stretching

I would stretch briefly before each workout—just a little bit. The way I did it was to spread all my fingers and my thumbs as wide as I could and then put my hands together in front of my chest, elbows out, with all the fingertips of one hand touching the fingertips of the other hand. Then, I would draw my hands in toward my chest. Once my hands were in this position, I could feel the stretch. The closer you push your hands together, the more stretch you'll get. Keeping my hands in this position, I would then rotate my hands like I was turning a big knob. The rotation plus the readily adjustable stretch really worked. Sometimes I would do this stretching during the workout, too, if I had to take a long break. I think you can see some of this stretching on my video. I also did a few wrist curl-style stretches, just to loosen up.

Always include a few regular full-range reps at the beginning of the workout with a gripper that you can close unassisted. These don't count on the scorecard (we'll talk more about that later), but should be included, along with some stretching.

The plans: what to do

"It ain't not knowing that's hurting ya, son. It's knowing so much that just ain't so." Having a plan is good. Having two or three is even better. Our objective is clear: hand strength with an unnatural level of crushing power. We want hands that are so strong, we're afraid to scratch ourselves.

This is like hunting that big buck deer. You've seen him and you want him. You know where he lives pretty much, but there's more than one trail he's using—lots more. You have to learn a few of them to have a chance: "He's never on this one during the rut. He uses these three in the mornings. Yeah, three. Whenever it's raining, he's in that thicket, but there's that other thicket where you saw some big tracks, and there's four or five trails going in and out of each of them." What are we gonna do?

Well, you could just get lucky and blunder into him one day, but me, I'm not that lucky. Better to have a few plans we can draw on to handle these different situations. This grip work will be a little easier than that wily buck—after all, you're in control of most of the situation most of the time. With two or three good productive plans to pick from, you'll be able to make progress under any conditions.

Some basic plans to consider are:

Training with hand grippers
You've got your full-range reps, forced reps, and negatives. You've got the electrical tape for high volume; you know all about the extended handle and about filing metal off the gripper handles to increase the range. That's pretty good variety for not much money.

First, let's make sure we understand what we're talking about with some of these terms:

Full-range reps – full-range reps are exactly what they sound like: the gripper is closed from the fully open position; then the gripper is allowed to return to the fully open position before the next rep is attempted.

Negatives – negatives are what would appear to be the part of the movement that we are stuck with, but not really what we're there to do. This, of course, is a giant misunderstanding. Let's look at closing the grippers.

When you close the gripper, you're on the positive side of the exercise. When you start to let the gripper return to its open position, you're on the negative side of things. It is here, during the return to the open position, that we have the opportunity to use a negative. If you just let the gripper fly open without resisting its travel, you have missed out. If you resist the gripper's return to its original position, you are doing a negative. When you use a gripper that you need to cheat shut, and you resist its return to the open position, you're getting into the best training there is.

Forced reps and assisted reps – they are the same thing and are done when the muscles are too tired to do any more work, but the workout requires more reps, or when you're training on a gripper you could never close unassisted in the first place. When you cheat a gripper shut, you're doing an assisted rep. When you put yourself into a situation where you're stuck with the negative side of the movement on a gripper you couldn't close unassisted, you're in a forced rep. We do these things to ourselves on purpose—they are not as horrible as they sound. The forced rep, or forced negative, is the same when training on machines: when you squeeze 385 lb. with two hands, and then let go with one hand, you're subjecting yourself to a forced negative. Have fun. This brings us to your next word, overload.

Overload – overload is using too much weight (more than you can handle) on a grip machine, or using a gripper that you need to cheat shut. This is how to get strong and will be explained in detail in the section on forcing adaptation. Please be patient.

Holds for time – holds (where you hold a gripper shut for a certain period of time) can be used when there is an injury you're trying to train around. It's hard to keep track of your progress when you're only doing holds, but they're better than doing nothing. When using holds for conditioning, you really don't keep score; you're just after the toughening up that the holds will provide to your skin and, most importantly, to the tendons. A bruised tendon can take weeks to heal. With proper conditioning these disasters can be avoided. If you're new to hard metal things being in your hands, you should consider holds for conditioning purposes.

Be negative: I'm positive it will help!
Do the negatives; don't be fooled by the naysayers. Negatives will help to make you stronger: whether you're using a grip machine or cheating out with a gripper and tape or the extended handle, the negatives work. When you're talking gripping muscles, you're talking small muscles. The best way to get these little fellers strong is to subject them to severe overload. Use the extended handle in the doorway, or just tape and guts, but give the negatives a decent chance. They worked pretty well for me.

When you're doing the forced reps with the extended handle on the gripper and the gripper stuck in the hole in the post, please pay attention to the following safety warnings I have for you:

1. *No tape—nowhere, never!* Don't use tape on the gripper handles when you do forced reps this way. The only time you tape is when you're training the normal way, without the homemade handle. When using the homemade handle, you want the knurling exposed to help keep the gripper handle stable in the heel of your hand. Besides, the only place we ever tape is the handle your fingers go on, and that handle is inside the tubing when you're doing this, so forget the tape. Trust me on this.

2. *Think about that wrist!* Stay alert. You must be constantly aware of the situation your wrist is in. When you're using a lot of bodyweight to cheat a gripper shut, you cannot allow any rotation of the handle inside the tubing or of the tubing in the drilled hole. There are a few ways to guard against this. They range from the high-tech (Stickum®) to the ordinary (pine pitch); you may need to use something, depending on the fit of the parts. Keep in mind that if the gripper flips one way or the other, you could injure your wrist. When you're doing forced reps this way, hold onto the spring with your free hand to prevent rotation of the gripper—which brings me to the next warning.

3. *Don't ever stick your thumb or any finger through the coil spring.* If you lose control and the gripper flips to one side or another, you could injure your thumb. Besides, when the gripper is being closed, the hole in the coil spring gets smaller. You don't want to be there.

Also, there's always the possibility that the spring on the gripper could break. When you hold onto the coil spring, *wear a good thick glove, like a heavy leather glove for protection*, because if the spring breaks, you don't want it to draw blood.

4. This is an easy one: *keep a clear head.* Don't let anyone distract you. Take that radio and do a weight for distance with it—or at least shut it off.

In plain words, it goes like this: I've done thousands of forced reps this way and avoided injury. *You've just got to pay attention to what's going on.* You're putting your wrist in a situation that could be dangerous if you're asleep at the wheel. Just stay alert; run everybody off is what I do. The thumb thing—I'm not kidding, if you insist on putting your thumbs in that hole, you need to have somebody take some nice photos of them right now, because they aren't going to look like that for long. If the gripper flips away from you, that thumb will be really long and sore. If the gripper flips toward you, that thumb will snap like a matchstick—the noise may bother your workout.

> **Warning!**
> **Never, ever put your thumb through the coil of the spring.**

Take it easy at first. Start with a gripper you can already close unassisted, just to get the feel of it. This is a good, comfortable way to get a high-rep workout that doesn't ruin the skin on your fingers since the handle extension is smooth. You're in business.

The gripper with the filed handle can also be used with the handle extension: just use it like a regular one, or you can use it with the filed handle exposed, and you'll be able to work beyond the range. With the benefits of the filed handle and the handle extension, you'll really be able to use heavier grippers than you normally would be using, and you'll be able to train beyond the range.

Training with a grip machine

Grip machines: if you have one, use it. It can be very helpful and produce a good workout. There are a lot of different types available, but whichever you choose, you'll need to figure out a way to do reps that make you stronger, not just tired. Pick one that will allow you to do overloads, assisted reps, and negatives. Do your shopping with this in mind. Use your imagination: even the most basic, primitive equipment can be helpful if you can figure out different ways to use it. A good example is the floor-model grip machine. It's been around for a while now—you know, the ones with the loading pins on each side or in the middle for the weights and the handles on top to squeeze together. Don't just do reps forever; load that thing up and squeeze it to the top, and then let go with one hand. This will leave the working hand with a severe overload. Even if you just hold it for two or three seconds, you're still getting more out of it than you would by just doing reps all your life.

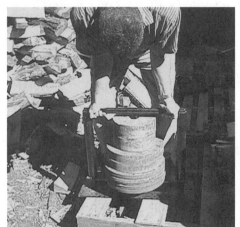

Joe Kinney doing holds on a Go-Really-Grip Machine.

But wait, there's more. What if you held it as long as you could and then fought it all the way down, as if your life depended on it? Well, I'll tell you what if. What you've done is a full-range positive movement, a severe overload hold, and a full-range heavy negative. Now squeeze it back up and repeat with the other hand. If you have one of those machines that costs big bucks, quit griping about the price. Use it this way and you'll get your money's worth out of it—and probably a lot more.

Work on a way to shorten the stroke when needed. A shorter stroke is just what the doctor ordered sometimes, especially when you get addicted to negatives. You'll want a pretty good range, but not fingertip range. I never did worry about the really wide open-hand position too much. I was not interested in gripping large-diameter objects. I just wanted to kill the grippers. When I did reps on my plate-loader, the positive movement wasn't even counted for anything on the scorecard: just the hold and the negative parts were counted.

Sometimes I trained on the grip machine by just doing more reps: when I reached 385 lb. on the plate-loader and didn't feel like doing more weight, I would just do more reps, only counting the negative, of course: 50 to 60 negatives with each hand, the base amount being 50, meaning when I did 385 for 50 reps with each hand, I would consider this "being up to 385 for 50 on the plate-loaded grip machine workout."

The next time I used the machine, six or seven days later, the workout would have to be 390 lb. for 50 reps or 385 for 55 reps. The next workout would need to be 395 for 50 or 385 for 60. When it gets up to 60 reps, I go up in weight, no matter what, and start over at 50 reps with each hand. After all, I've given myself an easy out for the last two grip machine workouts by just doing more reps, and now—time's up. Get real and add the measly 5 lb. and squeeze that thing like you want to hurt it.

Training with injuries
One important thing to know is what to do when you have injuries but you still want a grip workout. If the injuries are on the skin—torn calluses and splits—you're still in business. Just do cheat reps and holds for time. Holds for time can be used for conditioning and variety, or for when you're injured. They work just as well on grip machines as they do on grippers. They'll give you a chance to work the muscles while protecting skin injuries from most of the wear and tear that would normally occur.

Remember, if you're keeping score on your workouts (and you should be—weight, reps, tonnage—we'll cover that later), the holds-only workouts will be difficult to score. It's up to you to make sure that you're honest with yourself and to see to it that you get what you set out to do—or at least admit that you didn't. Only you know when you've done enough. Holds are hard to score and you're the scorekeeper. I hope we can trust this feller.

Workout schedule

My workouts were either with the plate-loaded machine or the grippers, rarely both at one time: I alternated the grip machine workouts with the gripper-only workouts. My schedule was weekends and Wednesdays: one gripper-only workout during the weekend and a grip machine workout on Wednesday night. You might do better mixing it up some and maybe involving more than one type of machine, or maybe doing some holds for time.

My gripper workout (with the extended handle) or my grip machine workout (with weight) pretty much followed the same pattern; I'll describe my gripper workout and you'll get the idea.

Gripper workout
During the weekend, usually at night, I would do a gripper workout that lasted anywhere from an hour to an hour and a half. There were days that I didn't feel too good, but what can you do? You can't hire somebody to get strong for you, so I did it anyway. Sometimes it lasted over two hours. I would do more weight or more reps every time—no matter what.

> "You can't hire somebody to get strong for you..."

Whatever you do, make sure you keep score: you need to know exactly what you did last time (I'll tell you how to keep score shortly). Assigning yourself a workload and making sure it gets done is what will guarantee your success. Without it, you won't be able to judge your progress. You'll start to think every time you get tired or start to bleed a bit, "That was pretty tough; that ought to be plenty. That was a good workout." I don't think so!

All my reps were done as singles, and no attempt to have a set and rep scheme was ever considered; only the total tonnage at the end of each workout was regarded as important. Take breaks as needed, but don't leave the area—you don't want to get distracted.

"What's tonnage?" you say. Let's take 385 lb. for 60 reps with each hand: that's a total of 46,200 lb. That's some tonnage, son, but hey, we're up to 60 reps now, so next time it'll have to be 390 for 50 reps; that's only 39,000 lb. What a relief. It's like a day off, isn't it? Soon you're up to 390 for 60 reps and your tonnage is up too, to 46,800 lb. This is the way to make gains, this is quite a total. Compare this total to your biggest workout, yes, even squats and deadlifts. Remember, we didn't even count the positive side of the movement when using the grip machine. Here we are at more than 23 tons, using what are probably the smallest muscles in your body ever to be targeted for exercise. We're blowing every other routine and total right out of the park. Maybe this is what's wrong with your squats and deadlifts and benches—just a thought.

Anyway, I guess you can tell I'm a firm believer in high volume and high tonnage. This was not as much fun as lying on the couch, but it produced a lot of strength. This was the only way for me. When I did low volume workouts, there wasn't much going on, but when I increased the volume, the strength just kept coming. Those of you who can make consistent gains with low-volume workouts should consider yourselves lucky. You've got it made.

A typical gripper-only workout would start with a brief warm-up and stretch and then just a few full-range reps with an easy gripper.

Next we go right to work on the grippers: slide the extended handle on the gripper you're trying to close and with the whole thing stuck in the hole in the wall, we start. Remember, just hold on to the outside of the spring (making sure that you're wearing that thick glove on your hand for protection). Now, using a combination of bodyweight and your grip strength, you cheat the gripper shut and hold for a count of two or three, maintaining a pretty good hold on the spring. Test yourself on every rep to see how much of the cheat (bodyweight) can be removed once the gripper is in the closed position. When you do release the gripper, don't relax your hold on the spring until you're almost to the fully-open position. Now, the other hand gets a try at it, same thing: one hand and then the other until you've done 50 or 60 reps with each hand.

You're forcing the gripper shut and holding for a good two or three count, hopefully, and of course working the negative side of the movement. At first when you cheat the gripper shut, you'll be able to get pretty good holds for time with each rep. That's the payoff: 50 to 60 reps, each hand, cheating it shut and holding. Of course, as the workout progresses, a count of one seems like a long time, and these hold times will decrease. Yet, every workout was my responsibility, so that every rep that wasn't good enough just wasn't counted. Take a break and try again. If you want real gains, you'll need to do real work. Eventually I was getting a three-count even on the last rep of the workout.

You reap what you sow. Sow good seed (real reps) and you'll reap a great harvest (stronger hands).

Take breaks as long as needed. Have a seat if you feel like it. I would sit down and goof off more at the beginning of the workout than I did toward the end of it.

You need to keep score on yourself, too. When I'm keeping score, I use hash marks instead of trying to write numbers. If you can get to the end of a workout and still write numbers, you aren't using enough weight. Load that thing up! Real reps with real weight—there is no substitute. Get over it. Just keep it very simple and very real.

Y'ain't mad, are ya? I don't mean to offend anyone, it's just important that you understand even though these training tips and tricks may sound good, the workload is still on you. You are the man who's going to move all that tonnage. More weight or more reps every time is the most productive strength-building recipe I know of. The downside is you'll probably bleed here and there, and you might see supper twice now and then. If you make big gains, you still win. Well, good, you haven't thrown this thing in the stove yet. I just figured you should know the reality of it. Now let's move on.

When working at really high levels of tension (or weight with a grip machine), it seems to me a slow start guarantees a better overall workout, so don't rush it and don't get discouraged if you start to feel tired early on. Take all the time you need. As long as you do more reps or more weight each time, you're getting somewhere. We're not pumping up for the beach here, so you don't have to restrict your breaks or any of that junk: this is about getting stronger. If you use your grip workouts to rep out on light to medium grippers, you will get pumped, but so what? The pump goes away and you're not stronger.

Meanwhile, I'm over here at my place taking my time and using the heaviest stuff I can get at the end of my workouts, and I don't have a great pump. The only difference that can be seen would be the occasional bleeding from under the fingernails. Who do you think is getting stronger?

Now you'll want to follow the same basic routine on your grip machine night, or mix up the two in one workout. It's up to you.

Scoring: good reps vs. bad reps
The workout might end up lasting more than an hour and a half. Only count the good reps. Let's compare the good rep, bad rep thing to something where we are not the judge and because of that, we can't cheat.

It's the end of summer and it's time to can beans. Your wife likes to do two loads at a whack because any more than that extends into the next day, and any fewer isn't worth the mess. Well, two loads is fourteen quarts and that's just about what one good bushel will make—a good bushel. Now, you could rush through there picking anything that looks like it might be a bean, but guess what happens when she gets them cleaned and starts working them up. She throws out all the bad ones. Then you're back out there picking more and you didn't really get too far trying to save time. You see, her finished product relies on both the amount of beans AND the quality of the beans. If you drag in another load of junk, she'll just dump them too. Only the good ones count—remember that.

A typical workout score sheet would look something like this. First you have your heading, and for me it was "No. 4 gripper with the handle and two-second holds" and the date. Then I had a line down the middle and hash marks down each side: hash marks in sets of 5 in a column of 12 (60 total), one for the right hand and one for the left.

After the work is done and you've reached your 50 or 60 reps, a long deep stretch is a good idea. You've done the job. You're guaranteed to get stronger because you're doing more weight or reps each time. You're getting what you paid for. It's time to leave your work environment and get back to your life. If you did it right, you won't have any mixed feelings. Don't linger, just walk away. We'll see you back here in a few days.

Hey, if you pick those beans right, you won't have any second thoughts when you walk out of there either.

Overall workout schedule
You should schedule your grip workouts in a way that not only gives you the time you need, but also protects your grip investment. These workouts will be more time-consuming than most. Plan on it. As far as protecting your investment, what needs to happen here is that any other workouts with exercises that tax the grip should be on days immediately after grip days. I think chin-ups and rows are worse than deadlifts when it comes to this. Maybe it's the long duration of a set of chin-ups. You might be hanging there nearly a minute. Your brain says, "Twenty-five chins," but your gripping muscles say, "One continuous long grip-destroying rep." Maybe it's the fact that when you're doing long sets of chins, your hands and arms are being starved of blood. Try weighted chins for fewer reps instead of a marathon set of 25. Most importantly, if you must do chins, do them on a day immediately after one of your grip days to give those muscles the most recovery time possible before your next grip day. You'll be investing a lot, so make it your business to protect it. All wrist curls, levering, and other

forearm work should be scheduled the same way. You might have to shuffle things around a bit for it to work out, but this scheduling thing is important and it's free. Take advantage of it.

Supplements

You're probably already on some kind of protein supplement, right? Or maybe just a high-protein diet made up of regular food? Well, that's just fine. What's good to know here is that you won't have to eat more tuna or slug down more protein shakes to increase or even double your grip strength. I'm not saying you don't need protein; what I'm telling you is that this job—even if your goal is to double your grip strength—simply will not require giant doses of protein. I did pretty well on regular food. The muscles involved here are small and they're going to stay small. My hands are so thick they look deformed, but we're still just talking ounces of muscle here.

The thing to keep in mind is that all of the muscles involved in this job, those in the hand and those in the forearm, don't amount to much in terms of muscle mass. The muscles that close a gripper are NOT the muscles that do wrist curls, reverse wrist curls, or any levering movements. The gripping muscles live underneath the big external muscles. The external ones move the hand in different directions. The internal ones close the hand. The ones that open the hand are somewhat exposed on the back of the forearm, but who cares? We're talking gripping here. When you close a gripper and all the muscles in your forearm seem to tense, it's only that they are doing their job supporting the position of your hand; they are not all working to close the gripper.

You won't need to eat three extra chickens a day to support this kind of development, so if you're already on a decent diet that has enough protein in it to support your other training, relax—you got the protein thing whupped. Myself, I'd eat those three chickens anyway, but that's just because I like them so much.

Seriously, though, with small muscles come small tendons and small ligaments. When you're training these little guys hard, they may benefit from some supplements. There are many supplements on the market aimed at joints and tendons, and minerals seem to be the key here. If you plan on taking your training to the outer limits of human ability (which is a place where I feel comfortable and enjoy being), you may want to consider a good mineral supplement to ensure the survival of your tendons and ligaments. I like the liquid ones best. I don't have to wonder if they are dissolving or not. Absorption is almost guaranteed, and I feel as if I'm getting my money's worth.

This stuff is all very boring to me. Let's talk testosterone—sure would be great to have more of that in you, now wouldn't it? But I'm not talking about some illegal stuff made for your horses. What I'm talking about here is the very best, custom-made test, formulated especially for you—no side effects, no jail time, your hair will stay on you, and best of all, you CAN afford it. Heck, you know if it cost a lot, I wouldn't have access to it. We want the very best and here's how we get it. What we're going to do on this one is to use a home brew. We can get the adrenalin level up to the danger point just by watching the news, right? Well, let's look at how to get the testosterone level up. So far the only muscles we talked about were the small ones. Now we need to involve the biggest of the big. We can use these big fellers to get the little ones what they need—the old squeaky wheel gets the grease thing. Nobody squeaks louder than the muscle groups used in squatting. No other exercise even comes close. Quit looking, it isn't there.

When squatting is used for the purpose of demanding a response from the body, the body gets the message loud and clear. The message must be urgent to get the best response.

If you've got the guts to do this, you'll be able to increase testosterone production starting tomorrow. Here's what to do: we're going to put the body into a state of emergency. Tomorrow morning, BEFORE breakfast, you will do squats. They can be done after you've charged up on coffee since it has no nutritional value, but don't eat ANYTHING: no orange juice either, no nutrients of any kind, got it? You need to go out there on zero nutrients to force the body to produce. If your body does not sense an emergency, there's no way it'll turn loose the hormones.

You'll be fine. Get out there and do a real squat workout—it won't feel good, but you'll live through it. Your body will produce the most testosterone it possibly can under these conditions. Make sure you use real weight in this workout. Your body will sense an emergency and produce whatever amount of hormones it thinks will be required to get out of this thing alive.

There is something to be said for "listening to your body," but it's not good. If you're in pain from injury or at risk of injury, you should listen to your body. If your body's just telling you it's tired or lazy, you're faced with a choice. Your body doesn't want to squat 400 x 20 for breakfast, but that may be what you need it to do so it'll produce. Under normal conditions, an adult man's body does not produce one bit more testosterone than the body needs to maintain itself. That's why we need the self-inflicted state of emergency: this will cause the body to release its reserve of testosterone for you. Every time you subject the body to this kind of trickery, the results improve. After a while of this kind of training, I could feel the increases in strength on a regular and predictable schedule. My body didn't want squats for breakfast, but my grip training needed the boost. I didn't listen to my body—I made it listen to me. Who's in charge here, anyway? If I listened to my body, I'd end up on the couch watching TV.

I like to do one long set of 20 to 30 heavies—yeah, that'll get things working. I would charge up on coffee and go get my testosterone supplement. Standing there in front of my homemade squat set-up, thinking to myself, "I can use this junk to make test, I want it and I'm taking it right now," I'd come up from the bottom so hard, the bar would bounce on my shoulders. You can't wait for life to send you the gains you want. Get out there and MAKE it happen. That's why they call it "making" progress.

The main focus of the stretching I used for the early morning squats for breakfast program was on the spinal erectors, with a lot of long and slow bending and stretching for these fellers, followed by a few make-believe squats. On the fake squats, I'd stay at the bottom position for a long time and really take it slow. This movement, along with the bending side to side for the erectors, pretty much took care of it. As I approached the bar, I'd throw in a few shoulder rotations and some neck stuff, and then it was time to go to work! I would do the first few squats slowly and build up to squats that would bounce the bar off my back. My squat workouts were for a very specific reason: I knew that was where the testosterone was coming from, and I made sure I got my full share every time. You notice the word "made" in there? You can't sit on your butt and wait for life to issue you huge doses of testosterone; you got to make these things happen. Good things might come to he who waits . . . some good things. Not testosterone, no. This stuff comes to he who busts his butt every morning while the rest of the world is still scratching itself. You know where it comes from—now get yourself some.

Everybody who joins the service does physical training before breakfast when they're in boot camp. They live through it. They do jumping jacks, push-ups, sit-ups, and they run. So don't worry: you'll live through it, with a good spotter, that is. You'll get better every time too. What you're actually getting better at here is making your body do what YOU want it to do and produce what you need. If you're already on a squat routine like this, meaning high-rep, very little has changed: you just do them on an empty stomach, first thing in the morning. An empty stomach in the middle of the day just isn't the same because you've been eating those chickens all day long, and your body's full of nutrients. Do it right, first thing in the morning. That way, you'll get the added bonus of daily doses of test, with free home delivery.

You won't miss out on the growing that we do squats for in the first place, either. You won't miss out on anything. As soon as you're done and can breathe again, you'll be right back in the house gobbling up breakfast, no problem. If you're not already on a squat routine like this, you're missing out. You've probably heard squatting makes you strong all over—well, they weren't lying. Testosterone makes you strong, and squatting this way makes testosterone. This is as simple as making mud, and it's free; get some. Get the *SUPER SQUATS* book from IronMind, and get strong all over.

The work ethic

Work pays, so we keep going there and doing it. Exercise, on the other hand, we tend to treat differently. There's a problem here and we're going to sort it out right now.

Nobody gripes and howls when their pay is short from taking days off. You worked less and you got less, that's fair enough. Why is it that these same folks act like they can't figure out what the problem is with their training? The answer is denial: nobody wants to admit they've been slacking off. They need to just get over it and quit trying to fool me. Most importantly, they need to quit trying to fool themselves. Your progress is akin to your effort and planning. They ARE a mirror image of each other. Unless you have a real physical handicap, expect no pity from me.

Look at training this way and see if it helps; remember, work pays and exercise just makes you tired. Let's say we have our next workout laid out, and it's going be a real killer. We need to do 60 forced reps using the No. 4 with the metal ground off the handle, each hand, of course. This could prove to be just plain horrible. You need to keep in mind that you're not putting out, you're getting. Don't look at this workout like exercise, look at it like your job, and if you don't do your job, you don't get paid/strong. Don't let anything stop you, because you know if you don't do it, you will not get paid/strong. I know you can do it. You might have a job you hate, but you keep going. This is really simple to figure out: this workout will pay, too; it will pay well.

The mind game

This brings us to the next subject, the mind game. Don't be scared of the mind game—you'll be in full control at all times. This is just another way to get our bodies to do what we want.

Try this one first: we can always hire somebody else to do it for us, right? Well, not really, but you can look at that workout and treat yourself as if you are someone else, someone who has been hired to do this job. Of course you are the one in charge, but just play with the idea and make believe the guy you hired is someone you really don't like too much in the first place: "Here's the job. Just get it done. No, I don't want to hear any of that," and, most importantly, "Nobody gets to leave until this is done." Treat it like work and it'll get done like work. This guy you hired (yourself) might gripe and howl a little bit, but so what? He works for you and you want this job done. Just put him to it and show no mercy.

The second one I call creating a state of emergency: this might not be good for your nerves or something like that, but I used it extensively throughout my training and haven't noticed any damage. Consider this: you're probably aware of the difference between your strength levels when you're relaxed and when you're furious, right? Well, don't be afraid to use a self-induced state of emergency during your training. Now, I don't want to read about you in the newspaper, so please go easy on this stuff.

I'm not telling you what particular thoughts I used to create this state, but you can be sure they weren't pleasant and it worked great every time. Everyone has something that will work for them, but here again, tread lightly in this area so you don't wind up committed or worse. Here's one that shouldn't result in any permanent problems: imagine you're rescuing someone from a really bad place. None of this will work if you're hanging out with the guys while you work out. Remember the section on the work environment? Here's where that stuff pays off. Now, you're rescuing this person in your mind and the only way to do it is to keep on squeezing this thing over and over. The radio's already been destroyed and you ran everyone else off, so it's just you and your time. Use your imagination and see what kind of state of emergency you can muster up.

This process has been taken to very high levels and the results were great. Sometimes I would work out so hard there would be blood coming out from under all of my fingernails by the time I was finished. I would keep myself in a state of emergency the whole time. Of course, this wouldn't be a good time to stop in and chat with me, but the work sure got done and the results were great. Yes, I was in a rage, but I wasn't screaming or anything. The guy who said, "Let it out, come on, talk it out," and so on was wrong! Don't talk it out, don't let it out. Use that stuff where it'll do you the most good: bring it to your workout and make a dent in the world.

The buffer zone: make sure you allow yourself a few minutes to cool off and return to the sociable feller you once were before heading back into the house. If you really get deep into this stuff, you may need more than just a few moments. Let that heart slow back down to normal. Running these little film clips through your mind in order to be the "psycho" grip guy is great, but don't subject your family to any of this stuff. These are your "tools" that you use to make great gains with. They are not dinner table material. Only you will know how many people you saved or how many bad guys you took care of during your little training session, and this is the way to keep it.

Forced adaptation
You can force your body to adapt. I know you can do it. You've done it many times before. This stuff isn't as mysterious as people would lead you to believe. We'll take a quick look at how it works, and you can build on this to suit your own situation.

Everyone has grown a callus or two in his life. This is an adaptation by your body to protect itself. You need to understand what the body is doing and what the body's priorities are if you want to have success. The body always tries to protect itself. When you feel burning pain from the sun, your body is telling you something: maybe time's up and you should head for the shade now. When there is a virus in your body, it doesn't take long to see how the body protects itself, trying to expel what it considers to be poisonous and harmful. Perspiring to cool off, eyes watering heavily in an attempt to protect themselves, and so on, there are many examples of this that we could review, but I think you get it. The best part of the body's priorities, the part we can and must exploit, is its insistence on restoring itself. This is a wonderful thing for the strength guy. You know the cycle: you shave, it grows back; the more you shave, the quicker it grows back—and thicker, too. So, we have the body's two most important priorities figured out: the body strives to protect itself and to restore itself. We can use these natural tendencies to our advantage. Remember, your body doesn't have the same goals as your mind does. Your mind wants to close the No. 4. Your body wants to be left alone.

Remember the old movie line, what we have here is a failure to communicate? The body sends us signals: I'm hot, I'm thirsty, I'm hungry. WE give it what it wants, but we fail to send IT signals so that it will give us what WE want.

Back to the calluses, you got lucky on them. Your body produced them because the danger of injury was obvious. Your body protected itself from your mind's idea of how much wood a man should split in one day. Do you realize what you just read? That's right. We're saying your body will adapt in order to protect itself from what the mind puts it through. We have the basic idea of what can happen, but what can we do to make it happen for us, in grip training or any other strength sport?

The answer is simple. We must communicate the correct messages to our bodies. One time my nephew was asking about my extreme training methods, and I told him, "It's like this: once your body is convinced that it will be destroyed if it doesn't start to get stronger, it will adapt. It doesn't want to adapt, but it's stuck with you. It may be convinced that you're insane, but it's stuck with you and whatever workload you think you need to do. When I do 60 reps with each hand, I'm really just after the last 5 or 10. You see, those are the ones that will force the body to adapt. They're the ones no human being has any business doing. All the other reps are just to get the body to that point, the point I like to call the bargaining point. This is where the mind and the body are doing battle. The body has communicated all of its messages by then: we're tired, we're sore, we're trembling, and all that stuff. This is where I win, because the mind isn't done working out yet.

"These last few reps are where all the gains come from because this is the part where the body thinks you'll surely kill it this time. But you don't, it doesn't die. It learns from this—not how to get stronger, it already knew how. It just wasn't going do it unless it had to! Now that it knows it could very well die from what this mind subjects it to, it has no choice but to adapt, and that adapting is what we call getting strong. If you're great friends with your body, you won't have much success. What you need to do is to put the body in such a state of emergency that it thinks it's the end, and do it on a regular basis. Twice a week works for me. My body is working full time trying to protect and restore itself. It never knows what's coming next because I always do more weight or more reps each time. It can't fall into a routine because no two workouts have ever been the same. When I say send the body a message, I really mean send the body a warning. A warning saying that it just gets worse, we're going to do more and more and more. Then it WILL adapt."

He didn't come right out and say he thought I was crazy, but that's probably just because he's kin.

The natural order of things

This little bit will be like an overview of what was just discussed, but still might be worth reading. The natural order of things just isn't good enough when what you're after is unnatural. It's not natural to be able to burst a can of beer. It's fun though. It's clear what we want is an unnatural level of strength; this is why extreme measures must be taken. Remember the work ethic: your results are a mirror image of . . .

You won't get too drunk eating corn. Somebody wanted to get drunk, though, and they used corn to do it. They mashed it, they strained it, they cooked it down, and they distilled it. When they were finished, you couldn't even tell what they started out with. Scaring the heck out of your body to force adaptation will not be the first time man has tinkered with the natural order of things. You can get blown up making whiskey. You might have a few tough days training, but the chances of being killed outright are slim.

Keep this in mind: if you listen to your body, you'll end up lying on the couch getting fat. If you make your body listen to you, you'll be much happier. Determination and guts don't come from books. You've got to rely on yourself for that stuff. You might be inspired or encouraged by something you read, but in the end, it'll be up to you. You'll be fine. If you've read this far and haven't thrown this thing in the stove yet, you definitely have determination and guts. I applaud you. Good luck in your training.

Examples of toughness
I used to know a man who could lift a 55-gallon barrel of diesel fuel into the back of a pick-up truck. He didn't do it for sport, he did it because his situation demanded it. At first he couldn't lift a full barrel, but after pouring and spilling, and pouring and spilling some more, over the years, he got to the point where he could lift these things so easily that it was boring to watch. He would knock them over and them grab them by the rims and clean them up to chest level. Before the upward momentum had stopped, he would give them a tremendous push forward (this part looked like a standing bench press). He had a lot of power and toughness.

Next, we have my old buddy Bob: this guy could split wood all day long. Regardless of the weather, you could count on him to be there and be ready—this was back in 1979–1980. We worked cutting firewood for pay. I would cut with the chain saw while Bob split. He would never stop to rest. He would literally split wood nonstop for more than an hour at a time. Once I got a bunch cut up, I would take over the splitting and Bob would start loading. The truck we used had a body that was 22' long, so trying to throw it in the end wasn't any good—you'd end up with a wall of wood right there at the end and still have to load most of it over the sides. The sides of this truck were more than 8' above the ground. Bob would kind of stagger around, half bent over, with one hand on a knee while he grabbed the wood with the other hand and threw it up and over the walls of the truck.

He'd switch hands and stagger back the other direction. This guy had a frightening grip and shoulders like basketballs—absolutely the wrong guy to wrestle around with. He never got to do 10 reps and then take a break; he got paid by how much he produced. You might say he got stronger by accident than most people could ever get on purpose.

Then we have "the tire man." If you get the chance to talk to one of these guys, make sure you shake hands with him: you won't be disappointed. Anyone who has changed tires on big trucks is strong. I'm not talking about pick-up trucks; I'm talking tractor trailer rigs and dump trucks. These fellers work their hands pretty hard. Yeah, they have the whole upper-body package if they've been doing it for a long time. Nobody told them to just do two tires and then take a break. They work eight-hour days doing this stuff. He's another guy you don't want to grapple with: he's always got a new injury and sometimes a short temper. You see, in these big truck tires, because of the loads, there's a lot of heat, and all the heat makes the tubes stick to the inside of the tires. These fellers have to wrestle the tubes out to patch them, which is tough work, and the tire man gets tough doing it. There are no days off to recover between every few sets. Non-stop hard work is life in the worlds of these men.

Setting goals and getting around roadblocks
Like a lot of things in life, goals can ruin you if you don't manage them correctly. Human nature and, in some cases, competitive drive tell us goals are natural and good. Once again, human nature is right: goals are natural and good. The problems start when goals are mishandled. Set them too high or too big, and you might end up miserable and frustrated. If you let yourself reach your goal, you're ruined. What we need here is something in between, something more on the line of a realistic starting point and the willingness to make steady adjustments. Here again, just like culling out the bad reps and keeping score, you will need to be brutally honest with yourself. Don't listen to that other guy. You know the one, the guy who's always trying to get you to take the easy way out. Yeah, that's him, the guy in the mirror. Big gains in strength rarely happen by accident. If you put your mind to it and plan for success, you'll have it.

The gripping game is tougher than benching or anything else where weight can be added in small, measurable increments. When it comes to goal setting on the bench, 330, 350, and 375 lb. are all legitimate bench press goals. With gripping, the space between the No. 3 and the No. 4 can seem enormous, and there isn't anywhere to stand. It's just space unless you can learn to create and manage goals. For example, there are a lot of different numbers between a 300-lb. bench and a 400-lb. bench, right? That's simple. Life is different with the grippers, though; you could completely master one and still just barely be bending the next one. Hmm, this IS different.

Well, there really are a lot of different steps in between, if you look for them. They're worth looking for, too, because they're so helpful in this goal-setting business. Looking at the void or space between the No. 3 and the No. 4, we can come up with a lot of different levels that we can use as stepping stones. Now we got some places to stand, places we can use to mark and measure progress. These steps can also be used when moving from the No. 1 to the No. 2 or any other step up, of course. Let's check them out.

List of adjusted goals, from the No. 3 to the No. 4
1. Kinney closes the No. 3 for the first time, and tells himself, "That's fine, but you sure didn't hold it too long." He's just then adjusted and set himself a new goal. This is simple, right? That's why it works, too.

2. He gets up to a 5 count on the hold, but, "Hey, what about your left hand? That ain't just for scratching yourself."

3. The right hand is good for a 10 count anytime. The left hand is now performing almost on demand, but is still not dependable. Even the smallest bit of progress is noticed though, since he times all the holds ands keeps score.

4. The left hand is good for a 5 count anytime now and the right hand is the dependable crushing tool I'd hoped it would be: "Hey, where'd you get this thing, out of a box of cereal or something?" Must be the testosterone talking. I paid for that testosterone by having squats for breakfast while the rest of the world was still scratching themselves. Let it talk a little.

5. From here on, things go pretty much as planned—because we have a plan. What about grinding the handles together? It's still tough to do with the left hand, but with the right hand it's really easy. This convinces me that I'm getting somewhere every time.

6. The left hand has grinding the handles as its goal. The new goal for the right hand is to slam the No. 3 shut so hard you can hear it clack together every time you pick it up. Don't forget to grind those handles.

7. Next we have the grippers that had some metal ground off the handles, remember them? They were discussed in the "Gearing up" section. If you made any of them, now is the time to use them. Remember, what we need are a bunch of little stopping-off points to use to prove to ourselves that we are making progress. Even though adding them in here now might make it look as if you're moving backward in closures and holds, you're not moving backward at all. You're really moving forward at a steady pace. This gives you many small goals between the level you're starting at and the level you're looking at.

8. Finally, and because that's the one I don't like to do, we have simply repping out. If you can use sets and reps to make progress and to monitor progress, they might be the right thing for you. Be creative and try to beat your last performance every time, even if it takes a longer workout.

Whenever testing yourself, it's critical that you give a hundred percent. You might feel worse physically afterward but you'll feel great mentally, knowing you've come closer and closer every time—and knowing that your workouts have paid you back.

Suddenly there are a lot of steps between the No. 3 and the No. 4, and we're not lost anymore. A No. 4 with the handle ground for more range can be a tough little monster. That's a good thing when you need it to add in here and there to keep yourself going the right way. You could use just the No. 4 and guts, but adding some ingenuity makes things go a lot smoother. All of these steps we went over can be done with the handle extension and then done again without it. You know the road now: small but steady steps.

Many of these little steps will be encountered during your regular workouts here and there: the cheats, the negatives, the holds. When used as stepping stones, they will be noted as steady progress, so you are never stuck at any level. You can claim success and progress just by adding a couple of seconds to your holds or by adding a rep here and there. These small gains might not seem like much to some folks, but when you're standing at the No. 3 and looking at the No. 4, you want all the encouragement you can get.

Only you can keep this thing going, so use every little stepping stone you can. Make constant adjustments to your goals. Remember the story about the mule chasing the carrot. He would walk all day chasing that carrot on a stick. If you ever let him get the carrot, he's done working and he'll stop walking. If you let yourself reach a goal, you will trick yourself into thinking you're done working. This is disaster.

Don't let this happen. You'll start to wonder what you're doing out here and why. It's critical that you constantly adjust your goals so that there's always a little bit more you need to do—not a lot, just a little bit, very small adjustments on a steady basis. After a while, you'll be able to look back and see that you've come a really long way, one little step at a time. Hey, that's how that mule was moving too. It just makes things go so much better when your goals are only a little more than what you're at now. Even if you think this is all fertilizer, you'll probably go through most of these stages anyway. Why not use them to help yourself?

That's why they call it making progress: you've got to make it happen. But, don't worry, you'll do fine.

A parting word

By now you've probably got a pretty good idea of what I think must be done to ensure success. All of what you've read here is based on personal experience: these things are real. They are not suggestions from someone who has "learned all about gripping" from the Internet. Watching someone run fast will not improve your speed. Watching me train will not improve your strength. You need to take advantage of the information that is being presented and use it to change yourself. The mind game information alone should be enough to make a big difference in your progress. Of course, this is only an opinion, but it's my opinion, and I think it's right.

Anyway this is the end of my section of the book, and we're about to part ways. You know I want the best for you. I'm not one to hide training secrets. What you've read is how I did it. The level of intensity at which you train might be different from where I was, but these are the techniques that I used. When these methods are combined with heavy doses of ferocity and determination, the results can be shocking.

I always trained at a high level of intensity. Working at the extreme outer limits of what my body could survive just seemed like the way to go. It didn't kill me, it made me stronger. Some famous old-timer said something like that way yon back in time. He was right. Of course, I don't want you to injure yourself; I just want you to know what has been done and to realize that you can do it too.

I would treat each workout as if it was mortal combat, a life and death struggle. Yeah, the intensity was definitely up there. I didn't "do" my workout, I went to war against it and never considered surrendering. I was the conqueror—every time.

Yet, no matter how strong we get, we must remember to humble ourselves before God, because compared to Him, we're still nothing. If you're inclined to, give this a try. Best of luck to you.

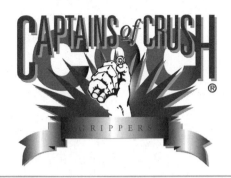

Chapter 7
The Holle Method for Training and Succeeding with the Captains of Crush® Grippers

by Nathan Holle

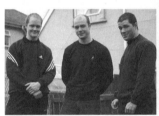

Nathan Holle (l.) and his brothers, Gavin (c.) and Craig (r.). Randall J. Strossen, Ph.D. photo.

None of us [Nathan Holle and his brothers Craig and Gavin] has ever done a warm-up. We don't think that there is any harm in a warm-up; it is just that we always just tore straight into our training. As the months of training have gone on, I now find that I need to remove the "clicks" and stiffness from my hands. Making a fist as tight as I can or closing the No. 3 does the trick. We would advise people to do the minimum warm-up they can get away with and still train at their peak.

If a gripper is easily within the reach of someone, then virtually any regular training will eventually get them there. Our current gripper routine takes about an hour: we train grippers three times a week, Tuesday, Thursday and Saturday, and sometimes we will train on Sunday as well.

I know it sounds a bit silly to tell people how to chalk their hands, but if you do it correctly, it can greatly aid your training (although some hands can perform just as well without chalk). Our technique on the grippers requires only the palm to be chalked (so that the fingers can slide over the handle), in a band across the hand at every point where the handle will be in contact with skin. Rub a little chalk into the hand and them remove as much as possible with a cloth, re-chalk before your first attempt, and then whenever you need it.

When you position the gripper in your hand, you are looking for a spot to anchor the handle securely, as far up toward the fingers as comfortable. If you make an open fist with your hand, you will see that the first bone of the fingers can only close to about a 90-degree angle to the hand. If the gripper handles are not closed when your fingers have reached this point, the gripper is never going to shut no matter how strong you get. In practice, the optimal position unique to you for maximum power could be a few millimeters closer, so that the fingers never make it to 90 degrees before the handles touch.

We place the gripper so that the bottom of the handle is on the first line in the palm just below the knuckles, and the top of the gripper handle is securely against the thumb pad. Also we place the gripper so that when we squeeze, we get all of our fingers as low down on the handle as possible for maximum leverage: only half of the little finger should be on the handle.

All of us find that loads of little things can help anchor the gripper, such as extending the thumb to stiffen the thumb pad and making a slight kink in the wrist. You will notice people get a better squeeze if they hold the spring or steady the handle with the finger: this is because the gripper is anchored much better.

When the gripper handle is in the best position in the palm, the other handle may be out of reach of the fingers, so you have to pull it in with the other hand. To keep the whole gripper from moving back out of position, press on the palm handle with the thumb of the other hand, so you are pulling the handle together with the spare hand using the thumb and index finger, and simultaneously squeezing with all but the little finger of the gripping hand. When you are "set" in the correct position, remove the non-gripping hand and squeeze in one swift motion.

When training, set the gripper very deep, that is, until the handles are about 5 mm apart, and squeeze from there. When you can close the gripper easily from this range, move on by setting the gripper a little farther out. It seems to us that as long as you can get some movement in the attempts, then you are on the way. We try to condition ourselves to give the attempt everything within a few seconds—finding that it is pointless to prolong the squeeze—so that you have completely given each attempt 100%. We have found singles, with a good few minutes rest between them, to be the way to go.

We do 4 to 6 attempts. This is based on good days and bad days (a bad day could be anything—an injury, feeling tired, etc.). Let's say you're setting the gripper to 10 mm but only moving it to 9 mm for the first 4 attempts; then there is little point in doing any more. However, if you are getting a good movement (say, down to 3 mm) on the gripper on the first 4 attempts, then go for 6 attempts. We try to limit the amount of singles to what is necessary. We have found using high numbers of attempts to be pointless, and you make yourself more injury-prone.

If people can't see a form of adding resistance or progression, they seem to be lost. In our opinion, the best form of progression is to develop the discipline to give every single attempt your all. To give an example of how all this comes together:

> **Chalk up (re-chalk whenever needed).**
>
> **Do one close of a gripper to remove "clicks" from your hand (or if you prefer, do a warm-up).**
>
> **Then using the gripper you are currently trying to close, set the gripper deep to about 5 mm and squeeze; take 4–6 attempts.**
>
> **Then using a gripper you can close: set the gripper as far out as you can close it and squeeze; take 4–6 attempts.**

> Do this for both hands. You should train the left and right hand straight after each other, so it is 1 attempt with the right hand and 1 attempt with the left and then rest, and so on.
>
> Once you can get all your attempts from 5 mm, next time set the gripper farther out. In our experience, when moving to a harder gripper, you can find yourself in a position where it can take weeks of training to go from setting the gripper to 5 mm at the start of the progression, to achieving a full +25-mm close. This is just as vital and just as productive.

Nathan shows the steps in training with partials on a Captains of Crush Gripper—in this case, with a No. 4(!):

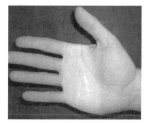
1. Chalking the hand.

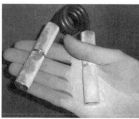
2. Correct placement of the gripper in the hand.

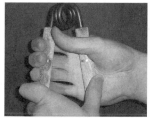
3. Beginning to set the gripper.

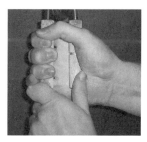
4. Setting the gripper to approximately 25 mm.

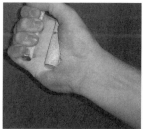
5. Beginning the squeeze.

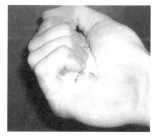
6. Closing the gripper.

It is not going to be easy and it won't happen overnight. We all have trained very hard and have tried many methods. Between us we have a combined knowledge of 10-plus years, and we have found that using the above training method has been the most productive and beneficial.

Below is one of Craig's recent training sessions; both hands are trained, but only the right hand is shown:

One close of the No. 3 to remove "clicks" from hand.

Attempts at the No. 4, aiming to set to 15 mm (all measurements made by Nathan and are all approximate):

Attempt	Set to	Squeezed to
1	15 mm	7 mm
2	13 mm	3 mm
3	15 mm	5 mm
4	17 mm	6 mm
5	19 mm	6 mm

Close the No. 3 as fast and as hard as possible but under control, aiming to set to 25 mm or above (all measurements made by Nathan and are all approximate):

Attempt	Set to	Squeezed to
1	30 mm	Closed
2	33 mm	Closed
3	29 mm	Closed
4	35 mm	Closed
5	30 mm	Closed

Duration of grip training: 63 minutes

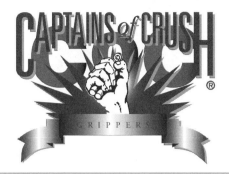

Appendix 1

Gripper Myths and Facts

Dog legs and seasoning: they are the stuff of some prevalent gripper myths, so let's take a quick look at them, burst some bubbles, and get you and your gripper training back on firm ground.

Dog legs

Myth

When a torsion spring is manufactured, one side has a slightly sharper bend where the arm of the spring feeds into the coil than does the other side, and elementary physics tells us with certainty that the force required to close the spring doesn't matter based on which of these two arms of the spring you hold steady and which one you push on. Nonetheless, some grip guys have been hoodwinked into thinking that it makes a significant difference which way they position the gripper in their hand.

Fact

Torsion springs are governed by a very simple law of symmetry: you can push on one handle or the other and the amount of force required to close the gripper is identical, which is why the idea of which arm of the spring is toward your thumb *machts nichts*. Incidentally, the same thing applies to right-hand versus left-hand springs: the direction of the wind will make no difference in the load required to deflect the spring.

Seasoning

Myth

What we call the "Tabasco sauce myth" is as superfluous as the dog leg fairy tale, although this time, even if just as incorrect, at least this concept could have a little zip to it. This false claim is that a gripper must be "seasoned," although the recommendation is not for Tabasco sauce or even a straightforward combination of salt and pepper, but rather a regimen of 50 or so reps, although some will put the seasoning level at 100 or more reps. Seasonistas claim that grippers start off "stiff" and that after a series of, say, 50 to 100 reps, a gripper will have become easier to close and then it levels off.

Fact

Once again, ignorance is the driver here because what we are really talking about is the spring bending when it is used: anytime a spring is overloaded (i.e., stressed beyond its capacity), it will deform (i.e. bend), just like a lifting bar. A sufficiently inferior spring will deform on the first rep, and a properly designed spring will never bend. Thus, a properly designed gripper doesn't have to be "seasoned" because it won't really change with use. On the other hand, the spring on an inferior gripper will bend (get easier) with use, which is why what starts with a spread of, say, 3" might shrink to 2-1/2" on an underdesigned gripper.

If this seems confusing, just think of lifting a bar, because the situation is analogous. Do you "season" your bar with, say, 67 reps before you go for a serious workout? Of course not. And let's go another step, by considering two very different bars: one is a generic bar made in China that you bought for about $100, and the other is an Eleiko bar, made in Sweden, that costs around $1,000.

Seasoning

Fact (cont.)

The first bar will bend the first time you load it to a few hundred pounds and drop it: and even though it might be called a "1500-lb." bar, see what happens if you try to load it up with anything close to that weight. On the other hand, the Eleiko bar can be dropped all day long from arm's length overhead with 500 or 600 lb. on it with no ill effect whatsoever and this is done all around the world every day.

Eleiko: The Story of an Unseasonably Strong Bar

To understand the myth of seasoning and the facts about bending, let's consider the lift that I dubbed "the Cholakov," in honor of the Bulgarian super heavyweight Velichko Cholakov, and run through an abbreviated version of a true story that was in the 2006 IronMind catalog:

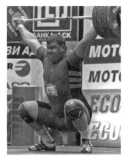 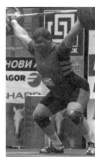 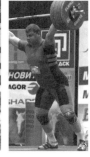 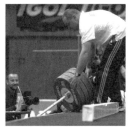

Going, going, gone! At the 2005 European Weightlifting Championships in Sofia, Bulgaria, Velichko Cholakov appears to have the barbell fixed overhead, but he eases into a forward lean, positioning the bar for the perfect two-armed put.

Velichko Cholakov stands about 6' 9" tall and weighs about 350 lb.; and in round numbers, he snatches about 450 lb., and he cleans and jerks about 100 lb. more than that. Consider a man of that height holding that much weight at arm's length overhead and, further, consider what has happened more than once when he was missing a lift. Instead of trying to guide the bar down, it's as if Velichko turns the miss into a two-arm put, but instead of a 16-lb. shot, we've got a 500-lb. barbell lofted on a terrifying trajectory in both height and distance. I dubbed this lift a "Cholakov."

One such Cholakov took place at the 2005 European Weightlifting Championships (in Sofia, Bulgaria). Velichko sent a missed 200-kg snatch flying right off the platform and the stage as well, so that one end of the bar nosedived to the ground and the other end was still up on the stage—a pretty severe drop for a barbell if there ever was one. I turned to Johan Erling, from Eleiko, and asked him, "Aren't you going to check the bar?" Johan answered with a quick shrug and shake of his head. "It's an Eleiko."

By way of contrast, one of China's top sets, Double Happiness barbells, were used at the 2007 World Weightlifting Championships, and by Jim Schmitz's count, the bars were replaced 7 times, even though there were no Cholakovs. And if they had been the really cheap bars from China instead of one of its most expensive sets, they probably would have been replaced much more frequently than this.

The point is that an inadequate bar will bend immediately when it is stressed beyond its limits and an adequate bar will never bend under conditions it was designed to withstand. It's the same with gripper springs. Going a step further, now you can understand why "heavy duty" grippers—coming from China and sold under different brand names—"season quickly," "keep getting easier," "just bend," "keep getting narrower and narrower," and so forth. They are like the lifting bar that really just doesn't have the strength to handle the amount of weight being put on it.

Captains of Crush Grippers, by being well-designed, are intended to perform like the Eleiko barbell described in the fall, and some other grippers, due to cost-cutting measures and poor quality controls, perform like the Chinese lifting bars.

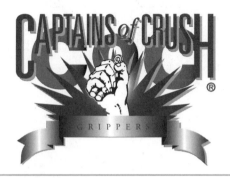

Appendix 2
Captains of Crush® Grippers: Rules for Closing and Certification*

Rules for Closing*

First, you have to be able to fully close a No. 3, No. 3.5, or No. 4 Captains of Crush Gripper according to the following rules:

1. The gripper must be an authentic IronMind Enterprises, Inc. Captains of Crush® Gripper.

2. The gripper cannot have been modified or tampered with in any way.

3. Chalk (magnesium oxide) may be used on the gripping hand, but rosin, tacky, etc. are specifically disallowed.

4. The free hand may be used to position the gripper in the gripping hand, but the starting position can be no narrower than the width of a credit/ATM card, and the gripster must show the official that he has an acceptable starting position by using his non-gripping hand to slide the end of a credit/ATM card in between the ends of the handles. Once

---

*The Rules for Closing and certification are subject to modification; please check our web site at www.ironmind.com for the latest details.

this is done, the official will give the signal to remove the card and begin the attempt. Any contact between the non-gripping hand and the gripper as the card is being removed will invalidate the attempt, and the non-gripping hand must stay at least a foot from the gripping hand at all times during the squeeze. Similarly, nothing may be in contact with the gripping hand or the gripping arm from the elbow down (for example, the free hand is not allowed to steady the wrist of the gripping hand or hold the spring, etc.). The entire squeeze must be clearly visible to the official: the gripper cannot be closed while blocked from view and then turned and presented as already closed.

5. The gripper must be held with the spring facing up.

6. The handles must touch completely.

How to Get Certified for Closing a No. 3 , No. 3.5, or No. 4 Captains of Crush® Gripper

You're able to close a No. 3, No. 3.5, or No. 4 Captains of Crush Gripper according to our Rules for Closing and you want to be certified. What do you do?

First, review the Rules for Closing (see above) just to make sure that you are closing the No. 3, No. 3.5, or No. 4 Captains of Crush Gripper under the proper conditions.

Second, please make sure that you can consistently close the gripper. If you have only closed it once, you may not be able to close it the next day, or more importantly, on the day you are to be verified by your witness. Wait until you have mastered the gripper, so that when you do close the gripper in front of your witness, all will go smoothly.

When you can close the No. 3, No. 3.5, or No. 4 Captains of Crush Gripper regularly according to the Rules for Closing and feel that you are ready to be certified, you will need to do the following:

1. Contact IronMind Enterprises, Inc. at sales@ironmind.com or at 530-272-3579 and let us know that you are ready to be certified. We will ask you if you can readily close the gripper and we'll take your name and address. We will then find a judge/witness who is in your area to verify the closing, and notify you of that person's name and contact information. This may take several days. You will contact the judge, who will be expecting to hear from you, and set up a mutually convenient time to get together. We will send the judge a brand new Captains of Crush Gripper for you to use for your closing. Your judge will open the gripper in your presence, and you are welcome to do a few warm-up reps on it before going for your close.

> Note: Please contact us only when you are ready to be judged—that is, please hold off if you are 1/4" away, or you maybe closed your gripper once, as we cannot line up your witness unless you are ready to be officially witnessed.
>
> Also, please do not line up your own judge as we will not be able to use the information. One of the ways we maintain the integrity of the certification process is by using objective, credible contacts to be witnesses.

2. Print out a copy of the Rules and Verification form (go to http://www.ironmind.com/ironmind/opencms/Main/captainsofcrush5.html) and take it, with a stamped envelope addressed to IronMind Enterprises, Inc., PO Box 1228, Nevada City, CA 95959 USA, to your verification. The witness will complete the form and return it to us.

3. You'll also need to provide:

   a. A photo (at least waist up) of yourself.
   b. A short bio, of a couple of paragraphs, telling us your age, weight, and height, where you're from, what your work and interests are, and something about your training and goals, and any other related accomplishments you would like to mention.

c. If you are a teenager, proof of your age with a copy of your driver's license, birth certificate, or passport, so that we may make a $500 contribution to the educational trust fund for Jesse Marunde's children on your behalf.

Send us your photo and bio either by e-mail (the photos should be in .jpg or .tif format) or by regular mail.

When we have received your signed verification form and the photo and bio, and they are all complete and in order, we will process your certification and feature you in the "Captains of Crush® Grippers: Who's New" section of the next issue of *MILO: A Journal for Serious Strength Athletes*. You will also receive your certificate, and your name will be added to the Captains of Crush: Who's Who list on our website.

Please let us know if you have any questions about how to become certified for closing a No. 3, No. 3.5, or No. 4 Captains of Crush Gripper—and best of luck with your training!

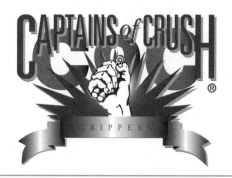

Appendix 3
Frequently Asked Questions about Captains of Crush® Grippers

Selecting a Captains of Crush Hand Gripper

1. Which Captains of Crush Gripper should I start with?

This is a little tough without knowing more about you, but generally speaking, we recommend:

- the **Guide** or **Sport** Captains of Crush Gripper for our younger and older customers, for women, and for anyone who hasn't really been training for strength

- the **Trainer** or **No. 1** Captains of Crush Gripper as the usual starting point for guys who have been lifting weights for a while: if you've been using sporting goods store grippers or specifically have been training your crushing grip, you'll probably want to start with the No. 1, especially if you have a gripper you can use for your warm-up; otherwise, a Trainer and a No. 1 would probably be best

Rarely, but occasionally, we will have someone close a No. 2 Captains of Crush Gripper the first time he tries it, and when we find this, it is usually someone who relies on hand strength as part of his daily work and/or is known for having a unusually strong grip.

2. How many Captains of Crush Grippers do I need?

We recommend training one hand at a time, so you can do all your training with just one Captains of Crush Gripper; but if you can afford it, we recommend that you buy two Captains of Crush Grippers, one for warming up (10 or so easy reps) and one for your work sets, ideally in the range of roughly 5 to 10 reps. If you would like to add a third Captains of Crush Gripper to your collection, we recommend that it be a half step or a full level above whichever one you can fully close—this is what we call your "challenge" gripper. For example, you might have a Trainer for warming up, a No. 1 that you can close for 8 full reps, and a No. 1.5 for singles or a No. 2 that you will use for partials, negatives, and holds.

Training with your Captains of Crush Hand Grippers

3. How should I train with my Captains of Crush Gripper?

Captains of Crush Grippers come with a training booklet, but our basic philosophy is to follow the general principles for building strength: train with very high intensity (as a percent of your maximum), using low reps and moderate sets. Many people train on Captains of Crush Grippers two to three times per week, but some train every day and some train as seldom as once per week. Some people like to do their grip training at the end of their basic workout and others prefer to do their grip training on their off days.

4. Captains of Crush Grippers are great for training while I'm watching TV, right?

Even though you don't have to change your clothes or go to the gym to train with your gripper, you'll want to take your training as seriously as if you were working on a big power clean, for example, so this is not something to do while you're driving, sitting at your desk, or watching TV.

5. When should I move up from one level to the next on the Captains of Crush Grippers?

Most people have to be able to do approximately 20 to 25 complete repetitions on one of our grippers before they can close the next level up, so we generally recommend that once you can do 10 to 12 full reps, it is time to start working on the next level. Joe Kinney, who certainly knows something about training on these grippers, would tell you to not even wait this long—he feels that doing negatives on a gripper one level above what you can fully close is the best way to make progress.

6. What should I do when I get stuck at one level?

The key principle is to add a new twist, so try varying your sets, reps, and number of training days. Try doing some negatives if you've only been doing positive movements. Try holds or partials if you've only been doing full-range movements. Use IMTUGs to attack your fingers one or two at a time. If you can't quite make it to the Captains of Crush No. 2, No. 3, or No. 4, give the Captains of Crush Nos. 1.5, 2.5, and 3.5 a try—they might be just the stepping stone you need. Try using a plate-loaded grip machine, such as the Go-Really-Grip Machine, and just as with a gripper, full-range and partial movements, positive as well as negative, are fair game.

And, most important of all, get inspired and knowledgeable by reading or viewing:

- *Captains of Crush Grippers: What They Are and How to Close Them, Second Edition* by Randall J. Strossen, Ph.D.

- *Mastery of Hand Strength, Revised Edition* by John Brookfield
- Grip training articles in *MILO: A Journal for Serious Strength Athletes*
- John Brookfield's "Grip Tips" at www.ironmind.com
- Blueprint for Grip Strength DVD by John Brookfield
- Grip Strength for Enhanced Sports Performance DVD, featuring Wade Gillingham

Remember to:

- warm up
- not overtrain
- focus on quality, not quantity, and vary your training to help keep your mind and body fresh

7. How do I integrate my Captains of Crush Gripper training with my other grip work?

If making progress on Captains of Crush Grippers is your main goal, training on them and doing related work on your crushing grip should be your top priority. Thus, do pinch gripping or any type of supporting and open-hand grip work after your crushing grip work or on a different day. It's the same with forearm work: do it either following your Captains of Crush Gripper training or on a different day. If you have trouble sorting this out, just remember the priority principle: do your most important training first, giving it top priority, and let everything else follow. This approach recognizes that you have only so much time and energy, so whatever you use for one thing will not be available for another.

8. Can you explain strap holds, negatives, forced reps, and partials?

Strap holds, invented by John Brookfield*, allow you to "add weight" to your gripper by attaching weight to a strap or belt; you then squeeze the end of the strap between the handles of the gripper, holding the handles shut for time or until failure. If you can't keep the handles shut tight against the strap, the strap and weight will fall. By adding weight, you can

*See "Handgrippers: Closing the Gap," *MILO: A Journal for Serious Strength Athletes*, July 1996, Vol. 4 – No. 2.

make it tougher to hold the gripper closed. Our Close-the-Gap Straps were made specifically so that you can train with strap holds.

Negatives, first used to great advantage by Joe Kinney in his training to close the No. 4 (see Chapter 6), are used to train on a gripper you can't close. Close the gripper using an aid (e.g., your other hand, your leg) and then remove the aid and hold the gripper shut with your training hand only for as long as you can, fighting to keep it shut until it finally forces its way open.

Forced reps are just that, continuing to do reps by cheating the gripper closed, pressing with bodyweight, your non-training hand, your leg, etc.

Partials are just what they sound like: doing reps by closing the gripper part way if you cannot fully close the gripper. You are moving from a fully open to a partially closed position; or from a partially closed to a fully closed (or more fully closed) position. Incidentally, don't confuse training on partials with doing deep-set closes as demonstrations or tests of strength. The former is perfectly legitimate and the latter is not.

These and other methods of training are included in this book, *Captains of Crush Grippers: What They Are and How to Close Them, Second Edition*.

9. I can close your No. 1 and have my sights set on closing the No. 2. What's your quick advice on how to get stronger on Captains of Crush Grippers?

Stay positive, be patient and persistent, and don't think of it as a little gripper—approach it the same way and with the same respect as you would approach a barbell loaded up for a heavy deadlift, so that you apply the same basic principles that work for developing all forms of strength.

Captains of Crush Hand Grippers—Care and Feeding

10. Your packaging warns about the risk of the spring breaking at any time. Does it really ever break?

Yes, but even though it's very rare on a Captains of Crush Gripper, we think it's important that you always train as if the spring will break at any moment. Let's explain this a bit. Anyone who has experienced breakage with the cheap imported grippers (whether with plastic or metal handles) or with an old Silver Crush™ Gripper knows how sharp the broken end of the spring is. The durability of Captains of Crush Grippers is something we have increased tremendously over the past 20 years, but for safety's sake and because safety is no accident, we always advise that you train with hand grippers—even Captains of Crush Grippers—as if the spring will snap at any moment. Remember this, too, when you train with IMTUGs, and be sure to keep your fingers on the handles, without wrapping your hand around the spring itself.

11. I live in Florida and I'm afraid my new Captains of Crush Gripper is starting to rust. How do I keep it as shiny as it was on day one?

Don't worry; the maintenance for a rust-free Captains of Crush Gripper is pretty simple. All you need to do is block moisture from the spring, so you can wipe it down occasionally with anything from a light oil, like WD-40, to car wax. If you prefer a durable protectant that also has a dry finish (unlike oil), give the Sentry Tuf-Cloth a try. Clean excess chalk from the knurling with a stiff nylon-bristled brush. That's really about all it takes to keep your trusty Captains of Crush Gripper humming along.

12. Is it cheating to put oil on the spring of my gripper?

No, absolutely not, but we appreciate that you are being so conscientious about this.

13. I like crickets and all, but my gripper is sounding like one. Is it defective? Can I do anything about it?

Not to worry: sometimes the edges of the coils on the spring rub against each other in just the perfect way to produce a creaking sound; it's not indicative of a structural problem, but if you find the sound annoying or distracting, a drop of light oil should dampen or eliminate it.

Poundage Ratings and Hand Gripper Variability

14. What's the story on the poundage ratings?

Ratings on grippers aren't nearly as straightforward as, say, weighing a barbell, but here's a quick answer (this topic is covered here in some detail in *Captains of Crush Grippers: What They Are and How To Close Them, Second Edition;* if you want to read more about it, see Chapter 3). Years ago, IronMind realized what a morass it was trying evaluate grippers and who had closed what, so we developed a rating system for making sense of Captains of Crush Grippers. It worked better than we had ever hoped because not only did we end up with something that helped us make Captains of Crush Grippers even more precise, but it also gave our customers a way to understand how much tougher, say, a Trainer was than a Sport. Taking things to another level, Captains of Crush Grippers are so well-established worldwide that grippers everywhere are often described by how they feel compared to our Captains of Crush models.

15. My friend has a gripper that is supposed to be 150 pounds but it feels about like your Sport, which you rate at 80 pounds. What gives?

Your friend's gripper might simply have a convenient number attached to it, without its really being tied to any specific test or measure (this is why the cheap grippers made in China, for example, all have poundage ratings like 150, 200, 250 . . . the numbers sound good, but don't expect them to really mean too much). This confusion and abuse of poundage rating for grippers is why we don't suggest that the numbers we supply for Captains of Crush Grippers will correspond to other grip devices.

IronMind's Captains of Crush Gripper ratings are internally consistent, meaning that they will help you understand the relative difficulty of our CoC grippers (e.g., how tough the Trainer is relative to the No. 1). Plus, they are empirically based; that is, our ratings are actual numbers derived from valid and reliable testing procedures, but we can't make similar statements about the numbers on other grip devices.

On the other hand, don't worry too much about the numbers: no matter how good or bad they are, actually training with your gripper is far more productive than analyzing it to death.

16. Do your grippers get weaker with time?

No, so don't worry if your No. 1 Captains of Crush Gripper is feeling easier to you now—it's because you're getting stronger! What is mistakenly called "seasoning" by some people is actually a weakening with use, and it's a reflection of an under-designed gripper with a spring that is bending, which is why it's not uncommon for low-quality grippers to get narrower and easier as they are used. On the other hand, Captains of Crush Grippers hold their line for a lifetime of steady training.

Getting Certified on Captains of Crush Grippers

17. How do I get certified for closing the No. 3, No. 3.5, or No. 4 Captains of Crush Gripper?

Read our Rules for Closing and Certification for all the rules and information (at www.ironmind.com). Best of luck!

18. What is certification on the Captains of Crush Grippers?

In 1991, to recognize his exceptional accomplishment in closing our No. 3 gripper, IronMind decided to "certify" Richard Sorin, documenting his feat of grip strength and establishing it as a high-water mark for others to shoot for and try to match. We included Richard's photo and feat of strength in our 1992 IronMind catalog, and when John Brookfield duplicated Richard's feat in 1992, our gripper certification was off and running . . . although it would be another two years before Tyce Saylor joined the illustrious Richard and John on the world's most prestigious hand strength list.

IronMind's Rules for Closing and Certification procedures have been honed along the way to reflect the spirit of legitimately closing a Captains of Crush Gripper, and over the years, IronMind has been what Richard Sorin calls "the good steward," guarding the strictness and fairness of this process. Anyone can jump on the bandwagon with a me-too product made in China and a me-too "cert" program on the Internet, but Captains of Crush Grippers have a unique history and rich tradition which set them apart, and this is reflected in the prestige of the Captains of Crush Grippers certification program.

Want to get on the list and earn the highest honors in the grip world? First, be prepared to train really hard and really smart, working your way up through the ranks of our benchmark grippers until you close the No. 3, No. 3.5, or No. 4 CoC according to our Rules for Closing. You'll then need to follow the procedure for certification.

What will it do for you? As with any goal worth achieving, the reward is in the journey and the knowledge that you did it right. Sure, you'll have the glory of seeing your name on the list of those having closed a Captains of Crush Gripper under certified conditions, but more importantly, you'll know that you can dig deep inside and with a big dose of dedication and persistence, and a measure of faith, you can climb the mountain.